EUROPEAN NURSES' LIFE AND WORK UNDER RESTRUCTURING

STUDIES IN PROFESSIONAL LIFE AND WORK
Volume 2

Scope

The series will commission books in the broad area of professional life and work. This is a burgeoning area of study now in educational research with more and more books coming out on teachers' lives and work, on nurses' life and work, and on the whole interface between professional knowledge and professional lives.

The focus on life and work has been growing rapidly in the last two decades. There are a number of rationales for this. Firstly, there is a methodological impulse: many new studies are adopting a life history approach. The life history tradition aims to understand the interface between people's life and work and to explore the historical context and the socio-political circumstances in which people's professional life and work is located. The growth in life history studies demands a series of books which allow people to explore this methodological focus within the context of professional settings.

The second rationale for growth in this area is a huge range of restructuring initiatives taking place throughout the world. There is in fact a world movement to restructure education and health. In most forms this takes the introduction of more targets, tests and tables and increasing accountability and performativity regimes. These initiatives have been introduced at governmental level – in most cases without detailed consultation with the teaching and nursing workforces. As a result there is growing evidence of a clash between people's professional life and work missions and the restructuring initiatives which aim to transform these missions. One way of exploring this increasingly acute clash of values is through studies of professional life and work. Hence the European Commission, for instance, have begun to commission quite large studies of professional life and work focussing on teachers and nurses. One of these projects – the Professional Knowledge Network project has studied teachers' and nurses' life and work in seven countries. There will be a range of books coming out from this project and it is intended to commission the main books on nurses and on teachers for this series.

The series will begin with a number of works which aim to define and delineate the field of professional life and work. One of the first books 'Investigating the Teacher's Life and Work' by Ivor Goodson will attempt to bring together the methodological and substantive approaches in one book. This is something of a 'how to do' book in that it looks at how such studies can be undertaken as well as what kind of generic findings might be anticipated.

Future books in the series might expect to look at either the methodological approach of studying professional life and work or provide substantive findings from research projects which aim to investigate professional life and work particularly in education and health settings.

European Nurses' Life and Work under Restructuring

Edited by

Jarmo Houtsonen
University of Joensuu, Finland

and

Gun-Britt Wärvik
University of Gothenburg, Sweden

SENSE PUBLISHERS
ROTTERDAM / BOSTON / TAIPEI

A C.I.P. record for this book is available from the Library of Congress.

ISBN 978-90-8790-980-2 (paperback)
ISBN 978-90-8790-981-9 (hardback)
ISBN 978-90-8790-982-6 (e-book)

Published by: Sense Publishers,
P.O. Box 21858, 3001 AW Rotterdam, The Netherlands
http://www.sensepublishers.com

Printed on acid-free paper

CONTENTS

PREFACE

The basis of this book is the European-wide research project entitled *Professional Knowledge in Education and Health: Restructuring Work and Life between State and Citizens in Europe* (http://www.profknow.net/). The project was financed by the European Union 6th Framework Programme, Priority 7, Citizens (Contract No. 506493). The overarching ambition of the PROFKNOW project was to understand knowledge "at work" among teachers and nurses as professional actors situated between the state, on one hand, and the citizens, on the other. Seven countries participated in the project: England, Finland, Greece, Ireland, Portugal, Spain and Sweden.

In this volume, parallel to the book on European teachers, the authors of the chapters use the outcomes of the project as a platform for further reflection on their research and to deepen their analyses. The focus is still on the changes in welfare states and restructuring of health care systems examined from the perspective of the nurses' experiences. However, the authors had the possibility to concentrate, from different theoretical approaches, on a specific problem area related to the main concerns of the original project.

There are many people whom we would like to acknowledge. First of all the project would not have been possible without the voluntary contribution of nurses and other health care staff in the seven participating countries. Regardless of their work load and hectic daily schedules, they were willing to participate in interviews and observations.

Many researchers have been involved in the PROFKNOW project, some of them directly in the research and others offering advice and commentary. They have all contributed to making this book possible. In particular we would like to thank Sverker Lindblad, who coordinated the PROFKNOW project, and Ian Perry, Principal Administrator at European Commission DG Research in Brussels. We also thank, in alphabetical order: Ari Antikainen, Jorge Ávila de Lima, Amalia Creus, Nasia Dakopoulou, Xavier Giró, Ivor Goodson, Fernando Hernández, Verónica Larrain, Erja Moore, Max Muntadas, Caroline Norrie, Ewa Pilhammar Andersson, Juana M. Sancho, Giannis Skalkidis, Areti Stavropoulou, Ciaran Sugrue, Dimitra Thoma, and Evie Zambeta.

We hope this book will provide new knowledge and insights not only to academic social scientists, but also to managers and practitioners working in the fields of health care and nursing.

Jarmo Houtsonen and Gun-Britt Wärvik
Editors

JARMO HOUTSONEN & GUN-BRITT WÄRVIK

INTRODUCTION

This book is about how European nurses' conceive their work and life in the midst of structural changes in welfare state, health care systems and nursing profession. Because our book focuses on nurses' experiences of and responses to structural changes, we need to locate nurses' work and lives within broader historical and social contexts. Therefore, as a background for the following chapters, we offer in this introduction a brief description of the globalization processes and the welfare state transformations, and how these are related to health care systems and the nursing profession. We also present some general methodological points that guided the research that contributed to this book. In conclusion, we summarize briefly the content of the book.

While we were editing this volume the world experienced a massive financial crisis followed by decreased investment, production and trade. No one seems to know yet how deep the slump will be before we move on to a new growth-track. Economic decline means that publicly financed welfare services are greatly strained since tax revenue falls. Consequently, health care systems may face new demands to cut costs and streamline. However, the current economic downgrade has also challenged the prevailing ideas concerning the organization and regulation of the capitalist free market economy. This ideological change might also bring about a disbelief in applying the market mechanism to the production and delivery of welfare services such as health care. For the moment we do have no idea about which way different countries may be heading.

WELFARE STATE AND GLOBAL CAPITALISM IN THE 21ST CENTURY

Welfare state and capitalism are closely connected. The emergence of the welfare state can be regarded as a compromise between class conflicts and distribution of prosperity and wellbeing among the various groupings of citizens in order to achieve a more equal society. Today, global economic competition is commonly used in policy discourse to argue for restructuring and trimming the welfare state so as to maximize cost-efficiency and utility for both capital and labor, or for both business and consumers. Some authors, such as Deacon (1997), have argued that welfare states are competing against each other, accompanied by international organizations and global discourse on supra-national policy issues, in order to regulate capitalism and protect the welfare services. However, if we assume that the welfare state provides a politically more or less neutral infrastructure for an innovative and competitive society, then there is a danger that we may not see the actual or potential

J. Houtsonen, G.-B. Wärvik (Eds.), European Nurses' Life and Work Under Restructuring pp. 1-13.

conflicts between capital and labor or between social classes or various interests groups in general. These conflicts are fought not only within states but also between states. The ambitions to abolish inheritance tax in many Western countries and the brain drain in the form of educated nurses from less-developed countries such as Malawi moving to the prosperous West are just two examples that illustrate how these conflicts cross national and international borders.

Koch (2008, 60-2) points to two important structural adjustments in the transition of welfare state in the face of trans-national capital accumulation at the turn of the 21st century. First, some of the authority in public regulation and decision-making previously held to the state has been increasingly taken over by, or given to, supranational bodies such as the UN, OECD, WTO, EU and World Bank. Second, the idea and practice of state regulation has changed from "government" to "governance". This means that there has been a delegation of authority to expert and non-governmental bodies and regional organizations, and the establishment of various public-private partnerships. In addition, the state does not so much monitor directly the welfare services provided by public organizations as it sets goals and benchmarking criteria and acts as a moderator and a collaborator between various constituents and interest groups. Moreover, voluntary associations and private firms are increasingly producing the welfare services for the "markets" where public organizations operate as purchasers.

The nexus between globalization, welfare state, health care and nursing profession can be approached from competing stances and projections (see Goodson & Norrie 2005). According to Brady et al. (2005, 923), so-called "welfare state reduction literature" holds that the transformation of global capitalism and the emergence of neo-liberalism as a dominant ideology have restructured the relations between the economy, society and policy and has rendered social welfare systems more feeble (see also Fairclough 2004; Mishra 1999). It is said that this transformation provides opportunities for the exploitation of uneven power relations between various fractions of society and threatens to increase the division between rich and poor people and nations. However, some argue that since globalization is also accompanied by global networks of human rights and justice, there are also discourses about the possibility of increasing, or at least protecting liberty and equality (Castells 1998).

Some authors argue that nation-states have become obsolete and have been taken over by multinational corporations and international and regional regimes (Barrow 2005). Others argue that the welfare states are just readjusting themselves in the face of global demands, and that welfare services are protected by strong interests and institutions (Esping-Anderson 1997). Still others, focusing on particular welfare institutions, see that welfare states are converging in the face of global demands, but only to a degree because of diversity in national strategies and historical path-dependent development (Antikainen 2008; Koch 2006; Mills et al. 2008). Consequently, many authors seem to believe that social policies tend to bow to markets and the exigencies of competitiveness (Koch 2008, 60). However, some empirical studies suggest that the harmful effects of globalization on the welfare state are not necessarily as strong and as all-embracing as assumed (Brady et al.

2005). The conclusion that can be drawn is that we do not yet have a complete picture of these structural transformations, their causes and outcomes.

When we look more closely at how these general welfare state restructuring trends are re-contextualized in health care systems in different national settings, we see that there is a strong emphasis on cost-efficiency, mangerialism and quality control (Dent 2003), which have impact on the organization of health care and nurses' work. For instance, Rafferty (1996) argues that 'new knowledge regimes' have emerged to manage and control the costs by means of health economics, evaluation and auditing as well as evidence-based medicine, clinical practice guidelines and health technology assessments. These influences are not confined to the Anglo-Saxon world alone, but have been at least partly adopted in many other Western countries as well. We should point out, once again, that there are national variations and path-dependent developments in health care policy and structures. Nevertheless, it seems that all states are trying desperately to balance their budgets and to adjust as competitively as possible to international corporations' efforts to globalize their profit-making and capital accumulation. This involves, among other things, tighter public spending and lower taxes, which both contribute to increasing cost-efficiency criteria and the rationalization of work in health care systems.

These structural changes put pressure on health care personnel all over Europe. In this book, we want to examine what happens to nurses' work and life when they are expected to adjust to these new demands. How do the European nurses experience these changes? Do they adapt or resist? The consequences of these structural changes in the working lives of nurses could be manifold. Kirpal (2003), for instance, suggests that one possible outcome is an increasing conflict between the professional identity rooted in the idea of patient-oriented care and the efficiency demands introduced by various managerial and organizational reforms.

STUDYING RE-STRUCTURING AND PROFESSIONAL WORKING LIFE

In this book, we do not focus on the causes of the structural changes, nor do we want to construct typologies of different countries on the basis of pertinent differences and similarities. Rather, we want to understand what happens in nurses' work and life in different localities when new restructuring measures are introduced in health care organizations. We also want to know how nurses experience and respond to these structural changes.

Restructuring refers to the changes in policy, regulation and administration of health care institutions, organizations and services. As we said above, the widespread neo-liberal and new public management doctrines and policies drive these changes causing some convergence in national health care systems. When we examine the local practices, we see that the processes and outcomes of restructuring vary across the national contexts. Even though there is convergence, perhaps due to the common driving forces of restructuring, different histories of each health care system and profession, and particularities of administrative measures and their implementation contribute to how this common trend refracts in each respective context, producing different outcomes at the level of various localities and nurses' everyday work (Goodson & Norrie 2005). Moreover, it is not only the calls for economic efficiency and professional accountability, but also the rationalization of administration (bureaucracy) and scientific and technological progress, and other societal changes, such as immigration and graying European population that contribute to the change in nurses' working life (Kosonen & Houtsonen 2007, 11).

Our book focuses particularly on professional life, work and knowledge from a bottom-up perspective. Consequently, we concentrate on practical and situational aspects of work and the issues that are meaningful for the nurses themselves without forgetting the broader structural changes. In the PROFKNOW project, we analyzed the issues that nurses talked about in interviews by means of a set of common themes including working conditions, control and autonomy, social relations, social position and status, education and learning, working-life balance and professional knowledge and expertise. By looking at the nurses' actions, perceptions and experiences from a bottom-up perspective in their respective localities, we want to analyze how restructuring measures are materialized, enacted or even resisted by nurses. Moreover, we aim to analyze the extent to which these measures are re-contextualized as new conceptions of professionalism and knowledge.

As mentioned above, there has been some convergence in the major structural changes in the governance, financing and labor management of health care in each country in the past twenty years or so (Beach 2005; Goodson & Norrie 2005; Kosonen & Houtsonen 2007). This convergence has not been universal or all-embracing in every sector of welfare (see Antikainen 2008; Koch 2006; Mills et al. 2008). But when we look at the general pattern of welfare state formation and change in health care, we can discern the following pattern. First, there was the establishment of universal, centralized and state-governed, and mostly tax-financed free health care systems. Then there was a noticeable transformation of the system due to neo-liberal trends of cost-efficiency, rationalization of administration, standardization of practice and accountability of professional work. However, the path and pace of this general pattern of change differs in each national case. Accordingly, we can talk about refraction of welfare state restructuring (Goodson & Norrie 2005).

In order to examine the differences between the countries, we divided them on the basis of appropriate properties into three groups. We were aware of the other typologies of welfare states presented in previous research (see e.g. Arts & Gelissen 2002, 143-4, 149-50). Because our main aim was not so much to distinguish between the types of welfare states, but to look at the nurses' working life from a bottom-up perspective we wanted to use fairly neutral typology. In this respect, the countries were classified into three types, the Offshore (the UK, Ireland), the South (Greece, Portugal, and Spain) and the North (Finland, Sweden) (Beach 2005). These categories correspond roughly to earlier categories of Liberal (Anglo-Saxon), Social-Democratic (Scandinavian), and Latin Rim (Late Female Mobilization), respectively (see Arts & Gelissen 2002, 149).

Even our simple classification is not without problems because each country has had its particularities in the welfare state trajectory. For instance, in the UK, liberalization trends started comparatively early on, in the 1980s, whereas the well-known socio-economic trajectory of Ireland has been unique. Nevertheless, in the literature, both countries are commonly placed in the Anglo-Saxon/Liberal category on the grounds of similarities in policies and institutions. In Finland, the welfare state began to emerge in the 1960s, picked up speed in the 1970s and reached its peak in the late 1980s. Restructuring measures were first introduced at the turn of the 1990s. As a Nordic welfare state, Sweden has preceded Finland in almost all these transformations. Finally, although Greece, Portugal and Spain were all under totalitarian regimes until the 1970s and only after that were welfare state institutions gradually introduced, they all have their national particularities.

As regards the neo-liberal and new public management policies and discourse, the UK has been at the forefront. Neo-liberal measures were introduced there already during the Thatcher era at the beginning of the 1980s. The Southern countries, on the other hand, have never achieved the scale of welfare services in the UK, Finland and Sweden. Nonetheless, there too some restructuring measures are striking. Finland and Sweden, for their part, have been relatively slow to adopt neo-liberal policies in any orthodox fashion. Furthermore, some special restructuring measures, such as contracting of staff, financing hospitals on the basis of results or rankings, or evaluation of process and outcomes, have had a profound influence in some countries but not others.

The transformation of welfare state institutions and professional organizations and practices is not, however, driven only by neo-liberal or economic concerns, but there are at least three inter-connected domains in operation. First, there is a neo-liberal ideology of free markets and economic efficiency. Second, there is an idea of rational management and administration. Third, there is modern medicine based on scientific evidence. These three domains all have their own principles, expertise and authority, which may also be antagonistic when the problems related to structures, policies and activities of health care systems are negotiated. Although these domains can be relatively independent they all are aspects of general rationalization and modernization of the West (Weber 1978) and therefore they may also often go hand in hand quite well. For example, formally rational administrative rules can be used to support the attainment of economic goals. Socio-technological management methods with ICT applications may make it easier to introduce certain efforts of cost monitoring and cost cutting. Evidence-based medicine can provide standards that are easier to relate to rational administration and economic calculation. It seems that at present, the economic domain with the neo-liberal interpretation of economy is dominating the administrative and scientific domains.

These changes mean that for nurses, caring and medical knowledge alone are not enough, they increasingly need administrative, managerial and even financial competencies in order to keep their organizations functioning and to maintain social legitimacy in the face of patients, colleagues, administrators and employers. That is, nurses' everyday working life is surrounded by medical (science), economic (efficiency) and administrative (bureaucracy) demands and expectations. These demands may come in varying guises, combinations and strengths in different national contexts. Furthermore, nurses may differ in their tendency and capability to recognize, activate or resist various demands and expectations. They also have varying resources and interests to adjust to or resist institutional calls for order.

General policies and discourses may still be rather distant from the everyday working lives of the nurses. Yet when these policies and discourses are being transformed into more concrete measures, such as evaluation and auditing of work, multidisciplinary health care teams or 'profit responsibility', they have a firmer bearing on nurses' work. In this book, we are mainly interested in those institutional changes that emerge as being influential or significant for nurses' working lives, identities and knowledge. Moreover, we focus on how structural and institutional forces are re-contextualized in the everyday working world of the nurses in various European contexts. Hence, it is possible that some of the restructuring measures are totally ignored by local actors or that local conditions and professional judgment produce outcomes that are contradictory to economic notions of efficiency, the administrative notions of rationality and the scientific notions of truth (Freidson 2001), or even public expectations of trust, communication and safety.

METHODOLOGICAL CONSIDERATIONS

When we try to analyze nurses' working life experiences in the context of the restructuring of the welfare state, we need to conceptualize the relation between social agency and social structures. At the level of working life, we think that it would be fruitful to view the process of re-structuring as an encounter between institutions and agents (Bourdieu 1981). Thus, we see nurses' work as socially conditioned practices that "bring together two states of history: objectified history ... and embodied history" (Bourdieu 1981, 305). Objectified history, or institutions, consists of rules, procedures and artifacts. Reforms in health care re-define objectified history and pose new expectations and demands with regard to nurses' work. The new restructuring measures are often objectified into texts, buildings and offices and are backed up by directives, job descriptions and training schemes. We understand embodied history as historically and socially formed dispositions pertaining to social agents' ethical, corporeal and cognitive tendencies, with an inescapable bearing on practice. Dispositions, acquired particularly in professional education and socialization, are manifested, for instance, with preferences for a particular job, styles for performing tasks, and in ways of dealing with equipment, expectations and job requirements.

Both institutions and dispositions are activated only if there is a reciprocal attraction between objectified and embodied history. Indeed, agents can work with institutional rules, procedures and artifacts only if they are inclined to do so as a result of previous experiences and training, or more precisely, to the extent and in a manner that their dispositions have been adapted to the institutional requirements beforehand (Bourdieu 1981, 2000). This means, for instance, that new efficiency measures such as evaluation of nursing are ineffective if they are not taken seriously by the nurses. Or, as Hargreaves (2005, 970-4) argues in the case of teachers, early career nurses are probably more enthusiastic and adaptable to change because they have been prepared for reforms in their training and have no experience of any previous change.

The health care sector consists of divergent institutionalized rules and procedures, belonging to medical (science), economic (efficiency), administrative (bureaucracy) and socio-cultural (patient) spheres that impose divergent mindsets on nurses' work. Different health care organizations and nurses are more or less well-prepared to adequately respond to the often inconsistent demands. In general, social agents differ in their tendency to recognize and activate the historical forces and logics embedded in institutions. There are different ways of experiencing nurse-hood since individual dispositions are formed in divergent social conditions through differentiated experiences and training. In addition, nurses follow varied trajectories and occupy distinct positions in health care systems with different resources, constraints and interests in adjusting to various institutional calls for order.

There are more institutionalized roles, functions and career paths for nurses today than ever before. There are, for instance, numerous medical specializations, and a division of labor between hospitals, primary care centers and teaching institutions and public and private care providers. It is practically a miracle that most individuals find their own place where they "feel at home" in this social mosaic. Collective expectations inscribed in a particular position and subjective hopes embodied in dispositions are usually in harmony due to various mechanisms of self-exclusion and co-optation in the training, recruitment and career of nurses (Bourdieu 2000, 216-8, 231-4; 1981, 308-13). For instance, the mechanisms of self-exclusion ('this is not a job for me') and selection ('he is the right type for this job') operate in the recruitment processes. There are, however, certain forces of social inertia inscribed in dispositions that may come to light when new expectations, introduced by institutional reforms, do not quite match the existing dispositions. Then, old understandings, aptitudes and skills seem to be passé or difficult to realize under new conditions (Bourdieu 2000, 159-61). This encounter between objectified and embodied history may produce various outcomes such as resistance, adaptation or disregard. These encounters – in the context of welfare state restructuring, changes in health care sector and nurses' work and life – are the focus of this book.

Although health care is organized by authoritative rules and we conceptualize practices as preconditioned by history and society, we try to avoid entirely deterministic accounts and leave space also for chance, strategic action and cognitive indeterminacy. There is always some room to maneuver, even in the context of standardized institutional and organizational prescriptions, such as clinical guidelines. In addition, jobs differ in terms of how narrowly and strictly they are defined and how much leeway is given to define rights and duties according to an officeholder's more specific likes and dislikes. Finally, the scarcity of resources may not make it possible to apply orders and guidelines at work. Indeed, the reality of institutional change cannot be found in the formal structures and static analysis of dispositions alone. Practical agents can neither create the principles and resources of their practices from scratch nor comprehend and control all the social, institutional or dispositional conditions of their practices (Bourdieu 1990, 126-7).

At a certain level, our book can be regarded as a cross-national study of nurses in the UK, Finland, Greece, Ireland, Portugal, Spain, and Sweden. This book in based on seven national reports and a common report on nurses' work and life (see Kosonen & Houtsonen 2007). The data on the national reports came from observations and interviews. We also conducted representative survey research in Finland, Ireland and Sweden involving 1,100 nurses and teachers in each country (see Sohlberg et al. in this book). A total of 4,519 individuals answered the questionnaire. The survey instruments and the variables are presented in the main report (Sohlberg et al. 2007). In addition to these reports, the project has also produced a cross-professional comparative report (Goodson and Lindblad 2008).

The study sites in each country were typical urban multicultural public health care settings where nurses interact with clients and other health care staff. We focused on two primary care settings and five hospitals. We selected three nurses from each country to participate in our study in order to have a representative of the following professional "generations": 30 years, between 8 and 10 years, and about a year of work experience. The national studies started with life story interviews to produce free flowing narratives of professional lives. These were followed by thematic interviews with a common set of themes, such as working conditions, work-life balance, knowledge sources, relations to colleagues and clients, and professional status and autonomy. Finally, ethnographies were produced by shadowing each nurse for three days at her place of work. In addition to this, the partners, except in Finland and Ireland, conducted focus group interviews with other nurses in order to further explore data obtained in the observations and interviews of individual representatives. Obviously, in our qualitative case studies, with just a few participants from each country, our data on nurses' work are limited. However, previous research reports from the PROKNOW project (Beach 2005; Goodson & Norrie 2005) produced extensive literature reviews, which offer us additional information that can be compared and contrasted to our findings.

There are two generic types of comparative study, which can be differentiated by the size of the sample, analysis techniques and strategies for generalization. First, there is the large-scale social survey that is analyzed by means of statistical techniques and generalizes on the basis of statistical significance. Second, there is the qualitative case study with few cases, and the generalizations of which are based on authenticity and credibility of results (Mills et al. 2006, 621-2). The application of qualitative methods to data analysis can be further divided into two types of orientations. First, there is a rather formal and analytical examination of data by using various tables and matrices. For instance, Ragin's (1987) Qualitative Comparative Analysis (QCA) of macro social events and processes belongs to this type. QCA tries to analyze necessary and sufficient conditions, measured as a constellation of dichotomous independent variables, with values 1 if an item occurs and 0 if an item does not occur in order to understand causal mechanisms that produce a particular outcome, which is also measured as a dichotomous variable.

Second, there is a less formal and more descriptive and interpretive understanding of the data, which we mostly employ in this book. For instance, Lindblad and Popkewitz (2003) ethnographically compare educational systems in eleven countries and show how classifications and categories for distinguishing people and social groups are constructed globally and emerge locally. This type of comparative understanding of cases does not, however, signify empathetic understanding or interpretation of intentions of agents. Instead, it presupposes contextualization of primary qualitative case data with secondary evidence, which comes in various forms, such as official statistics, professional and administrative discourse, previous studies and the immersion of the researcher in the socio-cultural context in which the cases are located. This type of understanding also depends on simplification and typification of cases as well. This means that each case that belongs to the studied set of cases is depicted so that only the pertinent characteristics are emphasized and in this way the case is assigned a distinguishable place within the set of cases. Naturally, the characteristics that best discriminate between the cases change when the topic and the focus of study changes. With this strategy, some of the richness and complexity of details is obviously lost, but by highlighting the most pertinent differences and similarities between the cases our understanding both of the broader forces, even at the global level, and the specific cases becomes more profound.

In the following chapters we will see that there are similarities and differences across the countries regarding how restructuring has changed the working conditions of the nurses and how the nurses have responded to these changes. However, we do not only try to typify our cases on the basis of pertinent differences, we also want to show what general outcomes are possible across Europe. Indeed, in line with Nermo (2000), we argue that important similarities can easily be overlooked when we are searching for differences in cross-national comparisons. Nurses' work, tasks and functions are to a large extent similar across Europe, as are the health care institutions, hospitals and health centers and their functions. Our descriptive approach to comparison is also intended to contribute to understanding the changes across the countries, instead of just bringing up the pertinent differences and leaving other details out by reducing the data to the features that distinguish the cases. Thus, we have tried to understand how the cases, on the one hand, converge especially due to global influences, and on the other, refract due to local particularities and histories.

ORGANIZATION OF THE BOOK

In the opening chapter, *The Socialisation and Commercialisation of Health Professions in Europe*, Dennis Beach discusses welfare state restructuring and trends in neo-liberal policy on a more general level, and with implications for health care and nursing. His point of departure is national case reports from the PROFKNOW project, but the scope Beaches' study is broader as he aims to analyze changes in the European service sector from a Marxist standpoint. He identifies a consistent pattern of similar processes of managerialisation, de-regulation, de-centralisation and rationalisation through standardisation in health care across the countries. The role of the state has been central in these processes of public to private transformation in production relations in health services and commodification of nursing labor power. Nursing has become productive labor that creates economic value and makes a profit. He summarizes the main restructuring tendencies in each country and argues that "nursing has developed as a practice that is increasingly organized and run according to basically equivalent neo-liberal standards, economic thinking and 'a Schumpeterian', market oriented open economy."

In the next chapter, *Nurses' Working Life Under Restructuring*, Peter Sohlberg, Magdalena Czaplicka and Sverker Lindblad analyze and compare the situation of nurses in Finland, Ireland and Sweden on the basis of PROFKNOW survey data. Their aim is to capture restructuring processes from the bottom-up perspective by taking into account nurses' opinions and attitudes as regards matters such as their education, working conditions and work organization. However, the authors also argue that restructuring cannot be captured simply by changes in numerical variables alone. They therefore develop an analytical conceptual framework with the ambition of contextualizing aggregate data in structural tendencies of the system-world (Habermas). In addition, they use the concept of organizational inertia, "based on the assumption that every organization /.../ have to handle the balance between stability and change," to analyze struggles concerning symbolic capital and uneven distribution of resources and power (Bourdieu). The outcome of structural changes is a growing demand for formal qualification of nurses and diminishing influence of professional knowledge. There is also a discrepancy between the subjective experience of control of work and the actual influence on decision-making.

The chapter by Beach relies heavily on the analyses of national policy documents (Beach 2005) whereas the analysis by Sohlberg et al. is mainly based on the survey data (Sohlberg et al. 2007). The next four chapters, on the other hand, originate from the national case study reports, which were based on ethnographic and interview data (Kosonen and Houtsonen 2007). The first three chapters compare all seven countries, whereas the last chapter focuses solely on Ireland and Sweden.

The aim of the chapter by Jarmo Houtsonen and Toni Kosonen, *European Nurses Articulating Care*, is to describe how the nurses in the seven PROFKNOW countries articulate the idea of nursing care. They discuss the diversification of nursing roles and work tasks all over Europe in recent decades. They describe nursing practices as being more varied across contexts, with ambiguities attached to nursing care against the backdrop of changing health care organizations. The nurses' perception of care is mainly two-fold, representing a division, although loaded with ambiguities, between instrumental versus expressive components of care. In addition, a parallel division between bio-medical and humanistic components was found in the nurses' talk about care, "reflecting the various epistemic sources of nursing science." Nursing is a dynamic configuration rooted in the changing organization of health care and division of labor between health care staff. Nursing is not just emotional labour or patient-centred care, but includes many technical, medical and administrative tasks too.

In their chapter, *New Management, Control and Autonomy*, Isaac Marrero and Jörg Müller discuss health care, nursing and New Public Management, which has introduced various measures of cost-control and accountability in health care. They analyze an apparent paradox between increasing professional autonomy and increasing professional control, and how such ideas have affected nurses' everyday work. Their argument is that the situation should not necessarily be seen as paradoxical but instead as a fundamental feature of a new professionalism created by managerial redefinition of autonomy and control. They also point out differences between the seven case studies from the PROFKNOW project in this respect. Moreover, they argue that nurses have gained more autonomy in caring tasks *doing* but have not gained control over administration and management *governing*.

The questions highlighted in a chapter by Helder Pereira and Constantina Safiliou-Rothschild *Emerging Work Transitions in the Nursing Profession* concern changing working conditions and how these are connected to nurses' definition of appropriate roles at work. They focus on problems related to health care restructuring expressed by nurses that cause stress and heavy workloads affecting both professional practice and working life. For instance, the shortage of time for nursing care, related to the shortage of staff, lack of resources and new administrative demands, has had a negative influence on nurses' professional identity. They also discuss new forms of employment contracting for nurses that are also emerging across Europe and the increasing entry of men into nursing, which seems to be changing the idea of caring. They conclude that in the present circumstances, nurses do not find conditions appropriate for working according to their professional ideals, such as holistic care and patient advocasy, because health care organizations do not share these ideals.

Finally, the chapter by Gun-Britt Wärvik, Rita Foss Lindblad and Maeve Dupont, *Patient Orientation of Nurses and Restructuring of Health Care,* discusses the consequences of health care restructuring for Irish and Swedish nurses by taking patient orientation of nurses as the point of departure. They make a distinction between relational, legislative and economic aspects of patient orientation and argue that these aspects should not be mixed up when analyzing implications of health care restructuring from the perspective of nurses. A conclusion is that economic incentives are attached to patient-orientation of nurses, linked to manpower issues in the Irish case study, and to nurses' documentation of their work with patients in the Swedish case.

To conclude, all the chapters discuss nurses and their work during a period of health care restructuring, both in terms of system narratives and life-world narratives (cf. Goodson & Lindblad 2008). That is, we want to understand nurses' experiences and reactions in the context of current changes in health care systems. Moreover, we want to show both the similarities and differences across the countries. The ambition of this book is to point to the general complexities and ambiguities related to nurses and their work, but also the unique situations in which these complexities and ambiguities are embedded. Our hope is that the book can contribute to the discussion of and research on the work and life of European welfare state professionals in general and nurses in particular.

REFERENCES

Antikainen, A. (2008). Power, State and Education: Restructuring and the Nordic Model. In J. Houtsonen & A. Antikainen (Eds.) *Symbolic Power in Cultural Context. Uncovering Social Reality*. Rotterdam/ Taipei: Sense Publishers, 85-97.

Arts, W. & Gelissen, J. (2002). Three Worlds of Welfare Capitalims or More? A State-of-the Art Report. *Journal of European Social Policy*, 12(2), 137-158.

Barrow, C. W. (2005). The Return of the State: Globalization, State Theory, and the New Imperialism. *New Political Science*, 27(2), 123-145.

Beach, D. Ed. (2005). *Work-package 2: Welfare State Restructuring in Education and Health Care: Implications for the Teaching and Nursing Professions and their Professional Knowledge*. Deliverable 2 in the EU Sixth Framework Programme Project Professional Knowledge in Education and Health: Restructuring Work and Life between the State and the Citizens in Europe. http://www.profknow.net/files/results/WP2.pdf. [Accessed June 2, 2008].

Bourdieu, P. (2000). *Pascalian Meditations*. Cambridge: Polity Press.

Bourdieu, P. (1990). *The Logic of Practice*. Stanford: Stanford University Press.

Bourdieu, P. (1981). Men and Machines. In K. D. Knorr-Cetina & A. V. Cicourel (Eds.). *Advances in Social Theory and Methodology. Toward an Integration of Micro- and Macro-Sociology*. Boston: Routledge & Kegan Paul, 304-317.

Brady, D., Beckfield, J. & Seeleib-Keiser, M. (2005). Economic Globalization and the Welfare State in Affluent Democracies, 1975-2001. *American Sociological Review*, 70(6), 921-948.

Castells, M. (1998). *The Information Age: Economy, Society and Culture: The End of Millennium*. Oxford: Blackwell.

Deacon, B. (1997). *Global Social Policy: International Organisations and the Future of Welfare*. London: Sage

Dent, M. (2003). *Remodeling Hospitals and Health Professions in Europe: Medicine, Nursing and the State*. New York: Palgrave Macmillan

Esping-Andersen, G. (1997). *Welfare States in Transition: National Adaptations in Global Economies*. London: Sage.

Fairclough, N. (2004). *Analyzing Discourse. Textual Analysis for Social Research*. Taylor & Francis e-Library. Digital book edition. (First published 2003 by London and New York: Routledge).

Freidson, E. 2001. *Professionalism: The Third Logic*. Cambridge: Polity Press.

Goodson, I. & Lindblad, S. Eds. (2008). *Cross-professional Studies on Nursing and Teaching in Europe*. Deliverable 6 in the EU Sixth Framework Programme Project Professional Knowledge in Education and Health: Restructuring Work and Life between the State and the Citizens in Europe. http://www.profknow.net/files/results/WP6.pdf. [Accessed December 15, 2008].

Goodson I., & Norrie, C. Eds. (2005). *A Literature Review of Welfare State Restructuring in Education and Health Care in European Contexts: Implications for Teaching and Nursing Professions and Their Professional Knowledge*. Deliverable 1 in the EU Sixth Framework Programme Project Professional Knowledge in Education and Health: Restructuring Work and Life between the State and the Citizens in Europe. http://www.profknow.net/files/results/Literature_Review_WP1_EU.pdf. [Accessed June 2, 2008].

Hargreaves, A. (2005). Educational Change Takes Ages: Life, Career and Generational Factors in Teachers' Emotional Responses to Educational Change. *Teaching and Teacher Education*, 21(8), 967-983.

Kirpal, S. (2003). Nurses in Europe. *Work Identities of Nurses across 4 European Countries*. University of Bremen: Institute of Technology and Education. ITB – Forschungsberichte 07/2003. http://www.itb.uni-bremen.de/downloads/Publikationen/Forschungsberichte/FB_07_03.pdf. [Accessed June 3, 2008]

Koch, M. (2008). European Statehood in Transition. In J. Houtsonen & A. Antikainen (Eds.) *Symbolic Power in Cultural Context. Uncovering Social Reality*. Rotterdam/Taipe: Sense Publishers, 55-66.

Koch, M. (2006). *Roads to Post-Fordism. Labour Markets and Social Structures in Europe*. Aldershot: Ashgate.

Kosonen, T. & Houtsonen J. Eds. (2007). *European Nurses' Life and Work under Restructuring: Professional Experiences, Knowledge and Expertise in Changing Context*. Deliverable 5 in the EU Sixth Framework Programme Project Professional Knowledge in Education and Health: Restructuring Work and Life between the State and the Citizens in Europe. http://www.profknow.net/files/results/D05_European_Nurses_Life_and_Work_under_Restructuring.pdf. [Accessed June 3, 2008].

Lindblad, S. & Popkewitz, T. S. (2003). Comparative Ethnography: Fabricating the New Millenium and Its Exclusions. In D. Beach, T. Gordon & E. Lahelma. (Eds.). *Democratic Education. Ethnographic Challenges*. London: Tufnell Press, 10-23.

Mills, M., Blossfeld, H.-B., Buchholz, S., Hofäcker, D., Bernardi, F., Hofmeister, H. (2008). Conversing Divergencies? An International Comparison of the Impact of Globalization on Industrial Relations and Employment Careers. *International Sociology*, 24(4), 561-595.

Mills, M. & van de Bunt, G. G. & de Bruijn, J. (2006). Comparative Research. Persistent Problems and Promising Solutions. *International Sociology*, 21(5), 619-631.

Mishra, R. (1999). *Globalization and the Welfare State*. Cheltenham: Edward Elgar.

Nermo, M. 2000. Models of Cross-national Variation in Occupational Sex Segregation. *European Societies*, 2(3), 295-333.

Rafferty, A. M. (1996). *The Politics of Nursing Knowledge*. London: Routledge.

Ragin, C. (1987). *The Comparative Method: Moving Beyond Qualitative and Quantitative Strategies*. Berkeley: University of California Press.

Sohlberg, P. et al. Eds. (2007). *Professional Expertise under Re-structuring: Comparative Studies of Education and Health Care. The Survey Study*. Deliverable 3 in the EU Sixth Framework Programme Project Professional Knowledge in Education and Health: Restructuring Work and Life between the State and the Citizens in Europe.

http://www.profknow.net/files/results/WP3_Final_report.pdf [Accessed February 11, 2009]

Weber, M. (1978). *Economy and Society. An Outline of Interpretive Sociology*. Vols 1 and 2. Berkeley: University of California Press.

DENNIS BEACH

THE SOCIALISATION AND COMMERCIALISATION OF HEALTH PROFESSIONS IN EUROPE

INTRODUCTION

This chapter is based on reading of a broad cross-section of investigations of restructuring in the service sector in Europe, particularly in education and health (e.g. Freidson 2001; Dent 2003; Edwards & Usher 2002; Robertson et al. 2002; Gordon 2005; Scott 2004; Sen 2005; Mahony & Hextall 2000; Jones 2005; Bernstein 2000; Lundahl 2002a, 2002b; Roussakis 1995; Beach, J. 2003; Woodward 1997; Warne & McAndrew 2004; Petronikolos 2003; Moutsios 2003; Nelson & Gordon 2004; Grollios 1999; Zambeta 2002a, 2002b, 2004 and Kazamias et al. 2002). However, it is focussing in particular on recently produced work package documents in PROFKNOW –project. (www.proknow.net; Beach 2005; Goodson & Norrie 2005; Kosonen & Houtsonen 2007). This research has highlighted several processes to be prevailent in each national case; managerialisation, de-regulation, de-centralisation and rationalisation through standardisation. Professional administrative autonomy and legal recognition of professional status are seen too, as aspects of professionalisation. These general trends have different manifestations in each country. Specific cycles of public to private transformation in production relations in the health-care sector and a massive movement of nursing labour into the private health industry as commodified labour power is also important and the research has also suggested that State involvement has been important in these processes. Conversions have occurred very recently in some cases and sometimes in very concentrated forms in others.

The processes of conversion also seem to be expanding in scope with negative consequences for professionals, professional(s') knowledge, professional identities and commitments, nurse-patient relationships and (in particular) the health-care services available to and consumed by lower-class fractions of health service recipient-consumers. As Kosonen and Houtsonen expressed it in their summary to Kosonen and Houtsonen (2007, 9-10), "calls for economic accountability and efficiency and the rationalisation of administration" have accompanied "neo-liberal restructuring in the health-care sector in general" and the nursing professionals and their practices within this sector. These trends refract a little differently in each country but they are common developments nevertheless, as "the contracting model of employment begins to dominate (numerically, administratively and ideologically) over the service model... Hospital, clinics and the health-care system… is now driven by demands for

J. Houtsonen, G.-B. Wärvik (Eds.), European Nurses' Life and Work Under Restructuring pp. 15-28.

increasing cost-efficiency, throughput and results, accomplished through guidelines, standardisation, evaluation and (extrinsic) rewards. For practicing nurses these... factors mean a (more) precarious career and tight resources that contribute to increasing experiences of workload and haste, stress and exhaustion."

BRIEF SUMMARIES OF NATIONAL DEVELOPMENTS SINCE 1960

Portugal

Nunes (2003, 320-321, in Beach 2005) characterises four main landmarks in Portugal: the establishment of a single basic training level aimed at providing general health care (1974); the autonomy of the nursing schools previously under the dependence of hospitals, that now came under the control of qualified male and female nurses; the single career of nursing professionals where all know their job and to which all have access (1981), as well as the integration of nursing education in the national university education system (1988). These changes empowered nursing professionals, most of which became civil servants with higher wages and lower working hours. To enter nursing courses, applicants needed a high school degree (11th grade). This requirement level was set due to a high number of applicants and led to the full integration of nursing education in technical college education in 1988. The nursing course (three years) conferred a bachelor's degree that enabled the first master's courses in nursing education to subsequently develop and a new career progression based on grades (grade 1 nurse, grade 2 nurse, specialist nurse, head nurse, supervisor and nurse technician made possible also by national regulations).

Since 1995 there has been a growth in regulation, by the consolidation of nursing education at the higher education level and by the introduction of new management models in hospitals and primary health care centres. This regulation clarified concepts and practices and characterised nursing care and practice as autonomous. It also functioned as a national regulation tool for the profession. In 1998 the Nursing Professionals' Association (Ordem dos Enfermeiros) was established, allowing the government to recognise nurses' aptitude for defining practice as well as for adopting an ethical and a disciplinary code that would assure the quality of nursing care.

From 2002 onwards, as a result of studies which indicated the need for more flexible management to increase effectiveness and also of some previous successful experiences, new hospitals were organised as limited companies or as private-public companies adopting management principles closer to private enterprise. That is, in this context, the State has the concession of the hospitals and primary health care centres and supervises the system. These hospitals remain within the National Health Service and its performance inspection system. The recent establishment of the Health Care Regulation Entity (Entidade Reguladora da Saúde) illustrates the State's growing role as a regulator in the field.

Ireland

The trends mentioned in the introduction of increasing professionalisation and increasing privatisation is clearly manifested in the Irish case studies in PROFKNOW. The evidence of increasing professionalism is suggested by the introduction of codes of conduct and the development of professional organisations as well as a move to academic education in 2002 with a degree programme being offered for the first time. This produced a substantial increase in theory and a proliferation of specialist posts and post-graduate courses. Privatisation in health services seems to have a detrimental effect on several aspects of quality of care. Professional education and training has also changed location over the past 40 years and a number of strategies will have to be introduced or enhanced before the expressed commitment to professionalisation can be realised.

The work of nurses is also undergoing change driven by the demand for a cost-effective, consumer-responsive service in line with the changing demographic and epidemiological profile of the Irish population. Marketisation is a fast developing phenomenon and has influenced the re-positioning of professional boundaries for nurses. This is evidenced by the introduction of the Scope of Nursing and Midwifery Practice Framework and changing forms of expenditure on in-service training since 1999 at a time of rapid socio-economic change. Moreover, the public health service is almost constantly reported as being in crisis with many patients awaiting hospital beds and waiting lists for surgery that are frequently reported as being unduly long. Private medical care is increasing and Irish nurses seek better career opportunities and remuneration in the U.S and the Middle East in particular. As a consequence in recent years, the Public Health service in Ireland has had to import nurses from the Philippines. It is amid this turbulence, which is set to continue, that new roles, responsibilities and career trajectories are being forged and the knowledge base of nurses is being re-formed.

Spain

The General Council of Nursing (Consejo General de Enfermería – CGE) is the organisation dedicated to the definition of the nursing profession and the defence of nurses' interests and health promotion. Its trajectory is therefore essential to understanding professionalisation, which is actually said to date back to the 16th century. Nursing was then defined as the 'art of healing', a conception that was in force until mid 20th century when the first Professional Associations (Colegios Profesionales) were born and the first attempts to develop a General Statute for nurses were made. It was not until 1978 that such Statutes were passed (Royal Decree 1856/1978), wherewithal nursing became a profession with a university degree recognized by the State and a Professional Association – the Organización Colegial de Enfermería (Consejo General de Enfermería, 2005). The Statutes were modified in 1993 (Royal Decree 306/1993) and completely redone in 2001 (Royal Decree 1231/2001) and 2003 (Act 44/2003). The nursing mission is now "to give health attention to individuals, families and communities during the full life cycle" through interventions based upon "scientific, humanistic and ethical principles". In 2003, the long pending definition of health professions was also accomplished (Act 44/2003).

The last milestone in the recent constitution of nursing on a legal level has been the Basic Statute (Estatuto Marco) from 2003 (55/2003 Act). The process of negotiation of the Statute was long and difficult. First drafts faced great resistance in several arenas of discussion. One of them was the competences: all nationalist parties considered that the legislation violated competence. Another issue was mobility. The plan to introduce the possibility of compulsory mobility was resisted and finally changed. In its final shape the Act conceives mobility as a right, not a duty, and it is rendered as voluntary. But again, some exceptions are allowed. The Act was finally passed with the abstention of the Socialist Party.

The altruist definition of the profession continues to be frequent ('help others'). But an economic discourse is emergent and nursing is now becoming more and more regarded as just another job, a way of making a living. This makes the social relations of production into a key question for nurses' professional practices. The dominant form of nursing is now a formally specialised hospital-based practice within a complex organizational system. A tight educational network allows for cohesion, a permanent flux of knowledge, collaboration, and the development of a professional identity. The trends of privatisation and professionalisation are again clearly visible in the Spanish case study materials (see particularly Beach 2005; Kosonen & Houtsonen 2007).

Greece

The welfare state deficit is evident in the low level of professional development in nursing till the 1970s in Greece, which was upgraded in the 1980s, the period of welfare state expansion that developed new opportunities and jobs for nurses. The universities were then perceived as the key to social status and upward mobility for professions and professionals. However, welfare state restructuring has taken place since the 1990s and has impacted on the profession in different ways. The profession is becoming more stratified and this is reflected in its internal organisation. Even though the state sector is still the preferred employer for nurses, there has been a substantial increase in the privatisation of health services in recent years, with adverse effects on working conditions. Professional burn out is a particular problem. Tensions are evident among a globally inscribed representation of quality as efficiency and evidence based policy and practice on one hand, and equality of access and democratisation on the other.

Between 1945 and 1974 there was no formal training before entering the workforce, and only 2-3 years of informal training at work sites. The profession was dominated by a medical discourse and the needs of medical practitioners. Nurses were simple assistants for hospital ward work. Between 1974 and 1989 a 4-year initial training was introduced along with Erasmus Programs and other EU collaborative efforts. No training was offered at work sites but the profession was still medically dominated. In 1983 Law 1404/1983 was passed regarding Technological Educational Institutions and the National Health Care System (1983) and in 1990 the first admissions to a Nursing degree programme at Athens University were made (1990). New curricula were established in 1995 and 1996. These were revised in 2003 and post graduate training was set up. Programmes for in-service training were also initiated in some hospitals. Autonomy of nursing professionals gradually emerged with the help of EU Directives of 1992, 1997, 1998 and the WHO directive 1992.

Finland

Up to the 1970s, policy issues that concerned the health care delivery system were mainly about building the service system and improving accessibility. The introduction of the Primary Health Care Act at the beginning of the 1970s formed the basis of the health care system and health policy. In the 1990s, developments in health care were influenced by 'external' circumstances: severe economic recession, the 1993 state subsidy reform, Finland's membership of the EU and socio-economic turbulence in neighbouring countries. However, a broad policy of preventive health care was still being pursued, whereby health was taken into consideration in all aspects of public decision-making. This extended developments from the mid-1960s onwards that put priority on health care and also shifted emphasis towards outpatient and primary care. In 1972 came the Primary Health Care Act and establishment of health centres together with the introduction of the national planning system. In the 1980s the health care and social services were incorporated into the same national planning and financing system and the Hospital Act in 1990 led to increasing deregulation and emphasis on municipal autonomy. About 10% of nurses now work in the private sector (Sohlberg et al. article in this book). Private hospitals and specialist practices are found in the bigger cities, particularly in Helsinki. Moreover, the number of for-profit nursing homes has been increasing in the past few years.

Estimations of the impact of restructuring on the nursing profession in Finland are vague. What is clear is that centralised steering was drastically reduced in the 1990s and the local administration's decision-making powers were increased. The development has led to a situation where the position and importance of evaluation has been strengthened. Evaluation is closely linked to evidence based practice, current care guidelines and health technology assessment at the national level. The cost-efficiency of the system is monitored carefully and the outputs of different hospital districts are publicised. Also apparent is that the education of nurses has moved from nursing colleges to the higher education sector, in the regional polytechnics 1990s. The duration of education has lengthened to three and a half years, and nursing science has been developed and established as an essential content of professional education. International standards have also been introduced. Postgraduate studies at the level of Master's and Doctorate Degrees are offered at some university faculties leading to administrative and teaching positions. Nurses have gained a stronger professional position in terms of education, knowledge and health care administration through their labour unions.

Sweden

Health care is often depicted as an organisation comprising three levels; primary care, county hospitals and larger region hospitals. Privatisation and market mechanisms have been introduced recently. At the same time as the state has parted with key economic governance tools in relation to detailed control of the municipalities. The 1990s is considered to be a period of extensive change in this respect in time with an economic crisis that reached its climax in 1992-1994 at the end of a short period of conservative government. However, the 1990s also witnessed substantial demographic changes as well as entry into the European Union in 1995.

Some key reforms are as follows. In the 1970s the so called 'Seven Crowns' reform was implemented. The reform stated that the patients would no longer pay directly to the doctor for outpatient care, but a fee of seven crowns to the hospital. This meant also that no private practice was to be carried out within the walls of public hospitals. In 1972 the county councils took over the district medical officers from the State and in 1982 a state commission (HS 90) pointed out the importance of preventive care. In 1992 The ÄDEL-reform was introduced. This reform implied that the care of long-term patients was transferred from county hospitals to the municipalities. This was an aspect of the decentralisation of the welfare state.

There were significant changes taking place in the beginning of the 21st century. For instance in 2003, an official report from a government committee (SOU 2003:23) stated that health care will never be able to fully meet all the needs of the citizens and that priorities will always exist. This report represents a retreat from the welfare state ambitions of full health care for each and every citizen according to need, established as an ambition in the "folk-home" project of the seventies. The committee also recommends that the development of health care should be steered toward open forms of care (i.e. in the home/family/community) and to preventive care. A variety of different private providers was also recommended but not for care that needs the heaviest technical and specialised resources of university or large county hospitals. These reforms have turned the emphasis of health care from inpatient to outpatient care, from hospital care to homecare and from a nationally owned and run public service to a more privatised organisation that emphasises and utilises the resources of (economic and rational) individuals and the family both 'practically' and discursively.

A Government Bill 1999/2000:149 presented an analysis of results of health care restructuring during the 1990s. The Bill explicitly gives the patients a more active position through an aim to further mobilise the patients' own resources. Patient involvement is not only for the benefit of the patient. On the contrary, the health care is outlined as dependent on patient involvement as a means to handle increasing demands. Patients are to contribute to the coordination of their own care and also influence its organisation and methods. Recent evaluations also suggest that municipal primary health care is an unattractive work place where access to doctors, nurses, assistant nurses, and rehabilitation staff is becoming increasingly limited. New personnel are constantly recruited. Long-term sick leave and early retirement is more common than 10 or 15 years ago.

England

Restructuring in England has had profound effects on the nursing profession, not the least in terms of objectification processes that have developed from the 1980s onwards in connection with an intensified economic management that has penetrated deep into the health-care sector. There is now a huge emphasis on target setting and auditing, with associated bureaucracy and paperwork in the NHS and the formation of 'new knowledge regimes' based on health economics, health services research and outcomes research. This form of audit culture started in the USA in the 1970s and it has reached levels of development in the UK that are not yet approached in any other European country. Its effects on the profession (professional esteem and self-esteem, professional identity, stress and burn out, biomedicalization of knowledge and the use of probabilistic knowledge to improve clinical performance) are the replacement of individual professional knowledge as the foundation for clinical decision-making and they seem to have been mainly negative. Other aspects are evidence based medicine (EBM), clinical practice guidelines (CPG) and health technology assessments (HTA). They have led to excessive paperwork that is said to be for quality assurance but which also plays a role in a culture of surveillance and blame.

In the UK it was suggested that nurses were once able to think of themselves as people within a vocational service, with a job for life, but this has changed considerably. The descriptions in PROFKNOW now suggest that nurses think in terms of nursing as commoditised labour; just a(nother) job. Moreover, new ways of thinking about illness and health have emerged. Illness, disease, disability, infirmity and care are new market opportunities and this significantly alters relationships between clients and nurses and the character of nursing work. Increased stress levels have accompanied these developments. A study by Britain's health and safety watchdog has found that nursing, dominated by women, was one of the most stressful of all professions. The Health and Safety Executive found that more than three in 10 suffered stress at work (Heath and Safety Executive, 2003/2004) and that people between the age of 41 and 50 were more stressed than older or young workers. Nursing has become increasingly marketised, individualistic and infused with an ideology of choice. Recruitment deficits, levels of stress and burn out and job dissatisfaction have intensified as has overseas recruitment. There have been no significant developments in education and training however in the past twenty years.

DIFFERENCES AND SIMILARITIES ACROSS NATIONAL DEVELOPMENTS

Descriptions like the above; which roughly refer to two kinds of development, professional knowledge and status on the one hand and privatisation and commercialisation on the other; may be taken to correct earlier suspicions from statistical survey research that there are different developmental trajectories in national health services and supply for the North, South and Offshore states in Europe, which are also said to be highly dependent on national contexts and politics. Because what is suggested in descriptions like the above, and even more clearly with regard to the national case-studies they are based on, is – as also Kosonen and Houtsonen (2007) suggest – that there are significant challenges to this idea of national independence and variation, particularly with regard to the new millennium. What is suggested is that there are significant consistencies (loss of autonomy, privatisation, commercialisation, fragmented professionalism, audit thinking, stress, burnout, retention difficulties, overseas' recruitment) with respect to present trajectories of change (http://www.profknow.net/fs-results.html).

Differences in health service structure and supply and the nursing labour process in Europe are particularly minimal from the turn of the new millennium and especially in the last three to five years, where nursing has developed as a practice that is increasingly organised and run according to basically equivalent neo-liberal standards, economic thinking and 'a Schumpeterian', market oriented open economy (Beach 2008, 2009). The EU innovation program, and its main development plan, the Lisbon Strategy, are based on such ideas, which imply a shift from national to post-national and networked modes of labour production and a new common concept of health care policy and practice within which national policy and internal professional demands are subordinated to the demands of an expanding European (or even global) market that employs economic competitiveness and increased privatisation as a motor of development. This kind of 'restructuring' not only changes the concept of welfare, it has a dramatic impact on working life as well, since it genuinely alters the definition of worker- and recipient rights and practices. New factors of professional culture are nursing for sale, illness as a market opportunity, flexi-labour and multi-tasking (Beach 2003; Gordon 2005; Scott 2004; Kosonen & Houtsonen 2007).

These things are common developments that are addressed in the current volume as are issues that are also identified in Kosonen and Houtsonen's work (2007), such as increased experiences of work overload and under-resourcing, increasing use of temporary contracts and stressful working conditions, reduced senses of autonomy, tightened levels of formal control and changing qualities in the characteristics of patient-nurse relationships. The following list summarises some of the main noted common developments.

- Decentralisation
- Development of an emphatic discourse of privatisation and marketisation (habituation)
- Company formation in the health-care sector
- Conversion of public health services to private interests
- Business takeover of ancillary services, health supply and nursing supply
- The creation of quasi markets for consolidating the processes of privatisation
- Authorities forming agencies for contracting out services to private suppliers
- Costs of administration shifted from ownership to managing and monitoring
- Increased costs from franchise effects (un/under-employment) on public employees
- The increased objectification of labour and increases in the value form of labour
- A dissemination of a view of patients as economically rational, self-interested consumers
- A redefinition of health-access and democracy in terms of consumer choice
- An increased objectification of health/ill-health and care-labour as factors of production
- Increased class differences in terms of supply and consumption
- Increased class inequalities in work conditions, contracts and education consumption
- Increases in judgement of performances according to consumer values
- Standardisation of care-assessment for comparison of performances

Restructuring in the health sector in Europe thus has a consistent pattern according to the PROFKNOW research packages and the chapters in the present book, even though this pattern is not exactly replicated in each country. Moreover, England is far ahead of the other partners in terms of the race toward full commoditisation. A number of things have been suggested as particularly noteworthy. These include:

- Three processes of development are ubiquitous instruments of change in relation to the restructuring of the nursing profession in Europe over the last 50 years (Beach 2009). These are (i) the socialisation and (ii and iii) the habituation and subsequent commercialisation of (professional) nursing.
- That in each nation involved in the research nursing and health are talked about and packaged (both in service supply and in education supply) very differently today than for 15 to 30 years ago.
- That we are also talking very much more similarly between national systems today than we were then and are also packaging health and health service training in similar ways as ‘travelling discourses and packages’.
- That education and training supply and development are rarely driven from centralist state monopolies, in for instance the universities or State bureaucracy, as in the past. Systems, people and events “outside” the (original) system seem to be pushing for changes far more than changes are pushed for and motivated from within.

- That the common trajectory of development through socialisation of labour power, habituation within the profession and its systems of education and training and a subsequent commercialisation and an influx of neo-liberal principles of governance is somewhat offset (time-wise) between nation states.
- That socialisation has principally almost always taken place in each country as a precursor to habituation and commercialisation, which can thus also be seen to prey on and socially, economically and discursively exploit publicly developed infrastructures, institutions, workers and practices (also Beach 2009).

This list is very different to the common description of the material contribution of commercialisation and competition to the development of an effective service infrastructure.

QUESTIONS OF GLOBAL CLASS AND GENDER

Within the chapters of the present book and in previous research accounts from PROFKNOW (see e.g. Goodson & Norrie 2005; Kosonen and Houtsonen 2007; Beach 2005, 2009) the issue of class differences has been suggested to be highly significant in the provision and consumption of health-care and nursing services. These class differences are historical and contemporary. They derive from issues of (economic) power and control through which the upper-classes in Europe have historically always been able to obtain private access to nursing and care from sources outside the home, such that the creation of common services there, in some kind of public model, represents a de-commercialisation of services rather than a movement from kinship systems to 'external' ones, as with respect to the economically less well off citizens. For them the creation of a common public system represents an externalisation of the domestic labour of women and the incorporation of this (predominantly female) labour power into public organisations (Beach 2009). However, what is also noticeable now is that neither process was ever fully secured in Europe (there were always parallel class-related processes of care going on) and that both developments are now anyway also being reversed in ways that show how global capitalism is significantly altering the relationships established in recent eras between social classes and the state in respect of nursing services. Interests of class parity have receded significantly as a direct result of neo-liberal insurgences into the service economy and have led to exacerbations of existing class differences (also Rosskam 2006; Beach 2005, 2009). In Europe today, although all sectors of the population avail themselves of an NHS (or its service-society equivalent) in a common 'national health interest', this is always supplemented from 'outside' the NHS and in two very different ways from for people of different class backgrounds. The level of supplement is on the increase, often encouraged by changes in taxation laws in member countries to stimulate individual responsibility and the private markets.

There are some important points here regarding the ways the welfare state national health concept in Europe should be politically, historically and economically understood. For what is suggested is that despite national rhetoric in some countries (such as Sweden) there has never been of 'one kind of nursing' in 'one system of health care' for all members of 'one classless state' equally. Nursing has always been (and is once again becoming increasingly) divided as a resource that is unevenly available and unequally distributed according to variables of social class, even though it must also be admitted that – through the stronger political organisation of the working classes, women and ethnic groups – a better material standard of nursing and health for all has been won in some countries (notably again Sweden) through struggles against the capitalist class and their political allies by trades-unionist and other folk-movements (Beach 2005, 2009).

Another key emergent point in the PROFKNOW -project that has not yet been discussed here is that nursing is principally, historically and contemporaneously, a female occupation that is increasingly recruiting candidates from lower- and lower-middle class backgrounds, or from low-GDP countries (http://www.profknow.net/fs-results.html). The processes of transformation that have taken place in respect of the formation of labour and the development of a (now increasingly commercialised) professional labour in the health sector are therefore principally referring to the successive movement of women's domestic labour. This movement of labour has been first from (lower-middle and working-class) homes to the public sector and then from public service to increasingly commercialised organisations as an aspect of economic labour power, where price-pressing (economic competition) and recruitment problems have now also led to increasing overseas recruitment as well. These are important points. They suggest that forms of (free) labour have been shifted into the broader arena of the production economy in a way that has implied both a feminisation of the economy and a potential ethical transformation of specific labour relationships on global-economic terms. This is usually said to have led to an increased freedom and independence for women. But this idea can be challenged through a material analysis of actual developments in economic terms, because this 'freedom' – if that is what it really is – has only been won at a significant cost.

Put very briefly the feminisation of the economy through expanded nursing labour has coincided with a less openly discussed general 'dampening' effect on real income levels for the lower and lower-middle economic portions in Western societies, with severe consequences for equality and liberty generally (Hill 2006), for which, with few exceptions, the social and material-economic situation of nurses is an example. Real hourly income levels for individual nurses have dropped significantly in the past forty years in Western Europe, on average, with the result that in general nurses have become low paid workers in relation to years of education and training who are incapable of supporting themselves and their families on a single income. Rather than the often spoken on freedom implied by liberal feminists through the explosion of women's paid labour in the public health sector, the development of this sector has actually primarily resulted in a more effective extraction of surplus value from production that is now, post-commercialisation, being openly exploited for economic profit.

CONCLUSIONS

The terms productive and useful labour, as discussed for instance in Marxist literature, become important concepts in respect of what has been suggested to have occurred with respect to nursing (as labour and as professional work) in the present chapter. In Marxist use these concepts differ from the understanding generally employed in bourgeois economic theory. Useful labour is a purposive activity which meets a human need. Productive labour is labour that is productive principally in the economic sense; i.e. labour that directly creates new economic value and 'makes' a profit for someone. It is the unpaid part of labour as measured in proportion to the total capital invested in production that is expropriated from workers and distributed by various means among the capitalist class. This is what I am suggesting has happened concretely, practically and theoretically with respect to nursing in the last 50 years.

However, there are also other implications. One of these concerns the role of the welfare state in the processes of capitalisation I am suggesting have occurred. Instead of being seen as 'the opposite' of private production and as an example of the redistribution of surplus value the welfare state becomes seen in this chapter as an intermediary in the creation of commodified labour power and the capitalist processes of conversion of 'other' value forms into objectively economic forms that are accumulated by capitalists through the sale and purchase of this labour and its products (also Beach 2009). In this sense, the expansion of the welfare state becomes an important intermediary in the growth of capitalism rather than something opposing and resistant to capital and commercialisation is no longer seen as a process that contradicts previous (social democratic/welfare state) developments of services and service values. Instead it utilises these developments directly in processes of accumulation of economic capital.

However, as also expressed in Beach (2009), this doesn't mean that the commercialisation and liberalisation of nursing doesn't embody an important political retreat from previous efforts to establish some form of social equality and democracy through health care provision. Indeed it does. The neo-liberal restructuring of nursing is dependent on an established material, social and knowledge infra-structure comprising people, places, tools, artefacts, technologies and practices. This infra-structure has often been supplied (and/or is currently being supplied) by public efforts using public resources to produce useful labour. It is now being 'privatised', liberalised and exploited for profit by private enterprises. The pathway of 'development' has been more compressed into the latter portion of the most recent decades in some countries (e.g. Greece and Spain), where socialisation and commercialisation are in fact operating almost in parallel, whilst in others (e.g. UK) developments have been spread over a longer time period and have progressed further.

REFERENCES

Beach, D. Ed. (2005). *Work-package 2: Welfare State Restructuring in Education and Health Care: Implications for the Teaching and Nursing Professions and their Professional Knowledge*. Second deliverable in the EU sixth framework project Professional Knowledge in Education and Health: Restructuring work and life between the State and the citizens in Europe. [http://www.profknow.net/fs-results.html]

Beach, D. (2008). The Changing the Relations between Education Professionals, the State and Citizen Consumers in Europe: Rethinking Restructuring as Capitalisation, *European Educational Research Journal*, 7(2), 195-207.

Beach, D. (2009). Socialisation and Commercialisation in the Restructuring of Education and Health Professions in Europe: Questions of Global Class and Gender, *Current Sociology*, (in press).

Beach, J. (2003). Professional Knowledge and Its Impact on Nursing Practice. *Nurse Education in Practice*, 2, 80-86.

Bernstein, B. (2000). *Pedagogy, Symbolic Control and Identity: Theory, Research and Critique*. Maryland: Rowman and Littlefield.

Dent, M. (2003). *Remodelling Hospitals and Health Professions in Europe: Medicine, Nursing and the State*. London: Palgrave Macmillan.

Edwards, R. & Usher, R. (2002). *Globalisation and Pedagogy: Space, Place and Identity*. London: Routledge.

Freidson, E. (2001). *Professionalism: The Third Logic*. Cambridge: Polity Press.

Goodson, I. & Norrie, C. Eds. (2005). *Work-package 1: A Literature Review of Welfare State Restructuring in Education and Health Care in European Contexts*. First deliverable in the EU sixth framework project Professional Knowledge in Education and Health: Restructuring work and life between the State and the citizens in Europe. [http://www.profknow.net/fs-results.html]

Gordon, S. (2005). *Nursing Against the Odds: How Health-Care Cost Cutting, Media Stereotypes, and Medical Hubris Undermine Nurses and Patient Care*. New York: Cornell University Press.

Grollios, G. (1999). *Ideology, Pedagogy and Education Policy. Discourse and Practice of the European Programmes on Education*. Athens: Gutenberg.

Hill, D. (2006). Education services liberalisation. In E. Rosskam (Ed.) *Winners or Losers? Liberalizing Public Services*. Geneva: ILO.

Jones, K. (2005). Remaking Education in Western Europe. *European Educational Researcher Journal*, 4(3), 228 – 242.

Kazamias, A., Zambeta, E. & Karadjia, Ed. (2002) Greece: Educational Reform 2000 - Toward a Paideia of Open Orisons - The Modern Greek Sisyphus. In S. Linblad and T. S. Popkewitz (Eds.) *Education Governance and Social Integration and Exclusion: Studies in the Powers of Reason and the Reasons of Power*. Uppsala Reports on Education 39: Uppsala University.

Kosonen, T. & Houtsonen, J. Eds. (2007). *European Nurses' Work and Life under Restructuring: Professional Experiences, Knowledge and Expertise in Changing Contexts*. Deliverable in the EU sixth framework project Professional Knowledge in Education and Health: Restructuring work and life between the State and the citizens in Europe. [http://www.profknow.net/fs-results.html]

Lundahl, L. (2002a). Sweden: Decentralization, Deregulation, Quasi-markets – And then What? *Journal of Education Policy*, 17(6), 687-697.

Lundahl, L. (2002b). From Centralisation to Decentralisation: Governance of Education in Sweden. *European Educational Research Journal*, 1(4), 625-636.

Mahony, P. & Hextall, I. (2000). *Reconstructing Teaching: Standards, Performance and Accountability*. London: RoutledgeFalmer.

Moutsios, S. (2003). The Identity of the European Union and the European Pedagogic Identities, *Comparative and International Education Review*, 47(2), 62-94.

Nelson, S. & Gordon, S. (2004). The Rhetoric of Rupture: Nursing as a Practice with a History? Nurse Outlook, 52, 255-61.O.E.C.D. (2001). *Education at a Glance*. Paris: Organisation for Economic Co-operation and Development.

Petronikolos, L. (2003). European Identity and Citizenship Education. The Case of Greece, *Comparative and International Education Review*, 47(2), 95-126.

Robertson S., Bonal, X. & Dale, R. (2002). GATS and the Education Service Industry: The Politics of Scale and Global Territorisation, *Comparative Education Review*, 46, 472-96.

Rosskam, E. Ed. (2006) *Winners or Losers? Liberalizing Public Services*. Geneva: ILO.

Roussakis, Y. (1995). European Citizenship: a symbol and a process in the New Europe, a challenge for Greece. In A. Kazamias and M. Kassotakis (Eds.) *Greek Education. Perspectives of Restructuring and Modernisation*. Athens: Seirios.

Scott, A. (2004). The Nurse: Autonomous Professional or Subservient Worker. In W. E. Tadd (Ed.) *Ethical and Professional Issues in Nursing. Perspectives from Europe*. New York: Palgrave.

Sen, K. Ed. (2003). *Restructuring Health Services: Changing Contexts and Comparative Perspectives*. London: Zen Books.

Warne, T. & McAndrew, S. (2004). Mirror, Mirror on the Wall, Who is the Most Improved of All? *Journal of Nursing Management*, 12 (1), 131-136.

Woodward, V. M. (1997). Professional Caring: a Contradiction in Terms? *Journal of Advanced Nursing*, 26(6), 999-1004.

Zambeta, E. (2002a). Europeanisation and the Emergence of Entrepreneurial Culture in Greek Education: Reflections from Education Policy, *Education and Social Justice* 4(2), 15-23.

Zambeta, E. (2002b). Greece: Modernisation and Control in Teacher Education. In E. Thomas (Ed.) *World Yearbook of Education 2002. Teacher Education: Dilemmas and Prospects*. London: Kogan Page.

Zambeta, E. (2004). Greek Education 1980-2001: From the Demand for Democratisation to the Promotion of Entrepreneurship. In Sakis-Karagiorgas-Foundation (Ed.) *Social Change in Contemporary Greece (1980-2001)*. Athens: Sakis Karagiorgas Foundation.

PETER SOHLBERG, MAGDALENA CZAPLICKA
& SVERKER LINDBLAD

NURSES' WORKING LIFE UNDER RESTRUCTURING[1]

> "The most important practical lesson that can be given to nurses is to teach them what to observe – how to observe – what symptoms indicate improvement – what the reverse – which are of importance – which are of none – which are the evidence of neglect – and of what kind of neglect" (Nightingale 1969 [1860], 105).

INTRODUCTION

In this chapter we will describe and discuss the situation of nurses in Finland, Ireland and Sweden. The empirical basis of this presentation is the PROFKNOW survey dealing with topics as, education, working-conditions, work-organisation and attitudes among teachers and nurses in Finland, Ireland and Sweden[2] When specifically relevant we will make comparisons with teachers in this chapter, but a systematic comparison between nurses and teachers is made in the survey report (Sohlberg et al. 2007).

In earlier studies within the PROFKNOW project (Beach 2005; Goodson & Norrie 2005) the focus has primarily been on general international trends of restructuring and their complex "refractions" within the national systems, i.e. the national, regional and local adaptations to these more general trends. From the empirical material in the survey, to be commented in this article, we have a complimentary and representative picture of what nurses actually are doing in their everyday-work and their preferences and attitudes. This presentation and analysis of nurses working life and experiences are made within structural contexts of different levels applying the concepts of Pierre Bourdieu and Jürgen Habermas.

The survey is the only method that allows for a generalisation of the results to the whole population, notwithstanding all paradigmatic and ideological criticism it could be exposed for. In the paradigmatic rhetoric about survey-technology it is often (partly correctly) associated with the universalistic claims of the positivistic

---

[1] The Profknow project has a cross-national and cross-professional focus. In order to facilitate cross-professional comparisons this chapter is written parallel with a corresponding chapter about teachers working life under restructuring.

[2] A majority of the items were construed specifically for the PROFKNOW project. However, in order to make relevant comparison possible some items were replicated from other studies (Wright 1997; European Social Survey, http://www.europeansocialsurvey.org/).

J. Houtsonen, G.-B. Wärvik (Eds.), European Nurses' Life and Work Under Restructuring pp. 29-58.

tradition where the goal is to formulate laws of universal applicability. When using the survey in the descriptive fashion applied here the aim is rather to show nuances and differences as well as general patterns. This is possible due to the comprehensiveness of the sample where various subgroups become discernible.

Nurses and Wage Labour

Seen in context of the high unemployment in Europe during the last decades it is clear that the position on the labour-market of Finnish, Irish and Swedish nurses is rather strong. A great majority of them (at least 80 %) have never been unemployed. The youngest generation, with the exception of the Finnish nurses, does not suffer of unemployment to higher degree than their older colleagues. For those who have been unemployed, it has been a rather short and isolated phenomenon.

Even though both occupational groups have a strong position in the labour market they differ when estimating their chances to get a similar job at another work-place where nurses are much more confident than teachers in their estimation of the chance to get a similar job.

A further aspect of the professional strength and organisation of an occupation is the degree of membership in trade-unions. This is particularly interesting as we have to do with nurses, highly associated with woman labour and an occupation earlier regarded as calling. A majority of the nurses are members in trade unions, but only a fraction of them (less than 10 percent) are working actively in the organisation. It means that the average member of the trade union does not participate in organised struggle for collective goals. A minor part of the nurses are member in professional organisations, but even this membership in a professional organisation is usually passive.

Voluntary work occurs outside ones professional obligations even though the professional skills are used. Although nursing originally was regarded as a calling only a minority of the nurses is performing voluntary work in the countries studied.[3]

Looking at the organizational context, more than 50 percent of all the nurses work in hospitals. About one of three nurses is working in primary health care. Other nurses are working e.g. in institutions, schools and company health care. One employer dominates the labour market totally as well for the nurses as for the teachers. The municipality or country council is the main employer for the Finnish and Swedish nurses and teachers while the Irish nurses and teachers are governmentally employed. Only one percent of the nurses are self-employed.[4]

[3] Only one of five of the Finnish and Swedish nurses are doing some voluntary work, compared with 1/3 of the Irish nurses. Neither do the majority of the teachers work voluntary, but compared with the nurses, they do this more often.

[4] About 10 percent of the Finnish and Swedish nurses and 20 percent of the Irish nurses are working in private profit oriented organisation or in non-profit organisation. Only 5 percent of the Finnish and Swedish teachers and 1 percent of the Irish teachers are working in corresponding organisations.

Nurses are wage-dependent employees and more than 60 percent work full-time and their everyday life is in an essential way structured by their working life. Expressed in other terms – an average nurse has been working in her occupation about 16 years. To work as a nurse is in general a long-lasting job with considerable experiences collected. The majority of the nurses live in a household with other people and in light of the feminization of the occupation this also should have implications for their general work-load, i.e. their practical working life is not exclusively devoted to nursing.

Almost all nurses are economically dependent on their wage-labour.[5] More than fifty percent of the nurses (between 53% and 69%) contribute to their households' income with at least half of the total family income.[6]

THE MULTI-LEVEL STRUCTURE OF NURSES' WORKING LIFE

The survey methodology comprising the empirical basis of this chapter is based on responses from individual nurses and we have so far merely discussed de-contextualized summaries of properties of the nurses as an isolated collective. In order to make the results meaningful they also have to be related to organisational and structural contexts. The perspective of the PROFKNOW project has been to capture restructuring processes via the everyday experiences of nurses and teachers, i.e. a bottom up perspective. This implies a complex framework with a variety of structural levels and positions' interrelating nurses actions and strategies with structural aspects. In order to capture the full range of changes and restructuring processes we also have to localize health-care in general as a social activity in a societal perspective and how it relates to governance and policy-making, the allocation of resources within the health-care system and the specific steering mechanisms applied. We thus have to cover the following aspects:

- The general localisation of health care as a social activity in a societal perspective and its position in relation to health-care governance, steering mechanism and the social fields of knowledge-production related to health care.
- The specific characteristic of the social field of health care e.g. internal hierarchies, and their relationship to adjacent fields, primarily academia and the medical profession. Furthermore a focus on what aspects of nurses' competence that is valued.
- The organisational structure of health care in the specific national case.
- The ideal-typical representation of nursing activities in interactional terms.
- A characterization of the concrete working environment for nurses in their everyday working-life.
- A description of individual resources, strategies, experiences and attitudes of individual nurses.

---

[5] A few percent in each group said that their earning only gives a small contribution to the shared household income.

[6] The corresponding share for teachers is even higher, approximately 75%.

From this list of aspects it becomes evident that the conceptual apparatus needed in order to contextualize the data must have a wide range. The catalogue of relevant characteristics could be greatly extended but the essential point is that every reasonable analysis and presentation has to take into account different levels. Important theoretically and for the following argument is that restructuring must be distinguished from mere change, even if this change would be big. Without assuming an essentialist understanding of definitions it is reasonable to regard restructuring as implying some sort of "qualitative" change beyond mere increase or decrease of numerical variables. The theoretical framework to be used in this study is composed of several structural models describing the relational "balance" or conflicts between elements or social groups. This could e.g. at different levels concern the ratio between market or public institutions or the hierarchical structuration of occupational groups or profession.

The health care system has gone through extensive changes in the last two decades. System changes can be described with structural concepts as "decentralisation, privatisation, marketisation, labour supply, secularisation, new public management and the use of information (IT)" (Goodson & Norrie 2005, 5). These are important characterizations in the vocabulary of the system-world. The question to be discussed in the following section is the relationship between these structural tendencies in the system-world and the experiences articulated with the vocabulary of the life world. What are then the implications of the multi-level perspective?

The bottom up metaphor applied in the project expresses the eternal division between actor/agent perspectives and structural perspectives (See e.g. Archer 2003; Bourdieu et al. 1991; Bourdieu 1984; Giddens 1984; Layder 2006; Mouzelis 1995). As a consequence we want to exploit perspectives and vocabularies within social science designed particularly to give a more substantial localisation of those positions.

The expression "bottom up" and the reverse "top-down" could in principle be used merely to depict the order of analysis and not necessarily to imply a causal order from structure to actor or vice versa. It is theoretically possible, though not the case within the PROFKNOW project, to use a bottom up perspective in the analysis even when adhering to a structural deterministic perspective where all measures of control and governance have an immediate impact. To illustrate this – we have in the PROFKNOW project used the metaphor "refraction" in order to express the idea that specific structural changes not necessarily have the same consequences in different contexts.[7] This is a trivial assumption concerning the pure formality of causal analysis, where causal effects always are dependent on specific contexts (see e.g. Ruben 1993).

The sociologically interesting aspect is that those different consequences of the implementation of similar policy measures in diverse national and regional[8] contexts

[7] One could argue that the metaphor "refraction" in itself implies something of a top-down perspective where the structural changes, coming from "above" are refracted in the "medium of everyday practice".

[8] In the Profknow project the regional context applies specifically to the Spanish case, where the regions have a high degree of autonomy.

to a high degree are related to the actual strategies and actions of the occupations studied.[9] These strategies could be characterized somewhere on the continuous dimension between adaptation and resistance.

In order to picture this complex situation we have chosen Jürgen Habermas' conceptualisation in terms of life-world and system-world and Pierre Bourdieu's idea of social fields. Habermas' perspective tries to capture the relative importance of different mechanisms of integration, or rephrased in more managerial terms, mechanisms of steering. This is particularly interesting for us in this context because the field of nursing represent areas where the relative importance of what Habermas regard as integration mechanisms, seems to be contested and controversial, i.e. we here have a tension or conflict between state and market as principal mechanisms of steering, as well as a tension between those two aspects of the system-world and the life-world (Habermas 1989). Another aspect of the importance of Habermas' normative differentiation between life-world and system-world is related to new modes of control related to "audit-society" where the reciprocal dialogue in communicative action could be sharply contrasted with audit (Jary 2002, 42).

It is necessary though not sufficient to picture the general relationship between the nurses and the system-world, represented by governing mechanisms of the market or politics. We also need as a complement a conceptual apparatus more specifically focusing on the intermediate level of nurses' working life and on their resources and how those are valued and used in the concrete setting.

In order to make more stringent some of the implications of the bottom-up perspective we would like at the intermediate level to use the concepts of practice and social field as formulated by Pierre Bourdieu. In a quasi-formal but substantial manner Bourdieu summarizes a conceptualisation of practice in the formula:

Practice = (Symbolic capital + Habitus) x Social Field
(Bourdieu 1984, 101).

There are several implications of this. In a negative sense it follows e.g.:

- Practice, according to this definition, is never directly observable but requires theoretical interpretation.
- It's impossible to get a full understanding of nurses' professional practice by solely concentrating on their individual and collective behaviour.
- Understanding of resources and the structural aspects can never give a full account of practice.

[9] The other principal factor has simply to do with that the different countries participating in the study represent different historical trajectories. Assuming that we experience an international trend towards New Public Management during the last decades of the 20th century the political, administrative and organisational milieu will vary e.g. between Finland and Spain and thus the result of the reforms, even with the (unrealistic) assumption that the reforms were identical.

In a positive sense it follows e.g.:

- The understanding of individual and collective behaviour should always be integrated with an analysis of resources.
- Resources or symbolic capital do not have absolute qualities but are socially determined within social fields. Within the social fields, that are hierarchically constructed there are conflicts concerning how characteristics should be evaluated as symbolic capital.
- Practice is composed of structural contextual elements as well as elements of actions.

To use as well Bourdieu's as Habermas' theoretical apparatus has some eclectic flavour to it. It could certainly be argued that, programmatic standpoints aside, there are fundamental differences in the respective conceptualizations of social life. Just to mention some aspects:

- Bourdieu is much more interested in hierarchies and struggles within the "life world".
- Bourdieu uses rather social field than all-encompassing notions as a structural concept on an intermediate/low level, implying conflicts of interests.
- Bourdieu is more oriented towards differences in the distribution of resources.
- Habermas has a much more general system-theory in an evolutionary fashion with stronger normative implications (Habermas 1989).
- Bourdieu lacks a systematic theory of the relations between various social fields (c.f. Leiulfsrud & Sohlberg 1996).

The rationale behind this pragmatic use of theories is to make a conceptualization possible of the grand picture of the general system level related to everyday practice (Habermas), without losing precision in the description of the intermediate level where the everyday life is structured by positions and actions within more delimited structures or social fields (Bourdieu).

We are in this context not interested in some kind of conceptual or programmatic fusion between the theories, but rather to use them as complementary structurations of the working life of nurses. Without going into exegetic details, the idea with using these rather different theories is that Habermas gives an overall view of important processes where the state and the market seem to colonise the life world, a macro-perspective lacking in Bourdieu. This is complemented by Bourdieu's conflict-perspective where he is interested in struggles concerning symbolic capital and the uneven distribution of resources and power as well as the systematic differences between individuals and classes concerning actions in terms of habitus.

Before applying Habermas' and Bourdieu's structuration principles, health-care could be localized within an even more comprehensive perspective, i.e. in terms of general functional localisation. Seen in the most traditional system-perspective health-care has to do with the "maintenance" of the social system, rather than being an active productive-force. In contrast with the situation for the educational system the health-care system is seldom regarded as an active productive force in the general discourse, nor is health-care associated with socialization aspects and normative reproduction. The discourse concerning the health-care system is often problem oriented, focused on increasing costs and demographic problems, though there also is a tendency to recognize progress in medical research and the developments of new techniques and treatments. Concerning the educational system we have discussed the balance, or conflict, between cognitive and socialization aspects for teachers everyday working life (Sohlberg et al. 2007). The situation for nurses is rather different as they are not part of a general socialization function, but there is an analogous balance (or conflict) between the technical curing aspects and the more empathic caring aspects of the work. The relative emphasis on either side could also to some degree reflect nurses' view on the relative importance of formal education vs. life experience, where a considerable part of the nurses regard life experience more important than education in their work-life. [10]

The functional view of health-care, tries thus to position the activity in terms of its general consequence and utility in a societal perspective. This aspect has lately been all the more relevant as we can detect an increase in the social engineering aspects of the health-care system. This increase is however not as dramatic for health-care as for the educational system, though the costs for health-care has increased rather dramatically since World War II. Health-care as well as education is an arena for ideological struggles concerning e.g. marketisation and the relative role of private or public institutions. In contrast with what is the case of education there are however seldom ideological conflicts concerning the internal and concrete work in health institutions.

We have here a profound change from latent functions depicted by the social scientist, to manifest functions intended by the policy makers. A simple indicator of this change of relative proportions between manifest and latent functions is the intensification of health-care reforms.[11]

We have chosen Bourdieu's conception of social field in favour of the more theoretically neutral concept of organisation. This does however not mean that organisational aspects of the health-care system on different levels are without informative value.

A crucial aspect for understanding possible discrepancies between policy measures on the systemic level and the actual situation in the life-world has to do with organizational inertia and this concept is applied below in analyzing our results. Taking into account that the policy-making measures have to be transformed in diverse organizational settings we have an additional systematic factor that could

---

[10] This is not self-evident as it could be argued that the empathic caring part of the job – in analogy with professions as psychiatrists or psychologists – also requires a formal education.

[11] This is not to say that all intended reforms (manifest functions) make the study of latent functions redundant. As the frequency of articulated goals and "bench-marks" increases those have however to be taken into account in the research.

explain the relative autonomy in the respondents' life-world that can be detected in our empirical material. This could be phrased theoretically in terms of organizational inertia based on the assumption that every organization (including educational) have to handle the balance between stability and change (see e.g. Ahrne & Papakostas 2002) The relative stability in view of the environmental pressure of change could then be seen in terms of the organizations' unwillingness and inability to change (ibid.).

A further organizational feature of relevance for us with implication for aspects of control and professional autonomy has to do with a specific division of labour within modern organizations. There are few modern organisations with a functionally uniform structure, either pure professional or formal "bureaucratic". More common is a double structure where administrative functions and professional knowledge are more or less separated. Health care institutions have generally this separation between professional and administrative functions. Nurses belong primarily to the professional staff, but they can, occasionally even be administrative leaders. It is the rapid development of administrative structures parallel or executive that makes new forms of control-mechanisms possible. From a general organisational perspective several aspects with important implications can be discerned for nurses. Both health care institutions and educational institutions could be characterized as open systems in the sense that they generally are tax financed and therefore under political control (see e.g. Scott 1998). The theoretical implication of this would be that they tend to develop traits of adaptability as well as measures of organizational inertia at different levels.

HEALTH CARE AND THE SYSTEM-WORLD

Habermas' conceptualization of the system-world is done in terms of what are the most general integrative mechanisms coordinating activities within the system. The mechanism characterizing the system-world and its integration is according to Habermas power (the state) and money (the market). Habermas contra poses those two mechanisms of integration with what he sees as the normatively ideal mechanism of integration, i.e. the communicative action (Habermas 1989). The relevance of this dichotomization of the system-world in terms of state and market is in this context that it reflects the main ideological cleavage concerning how the health-care system should be run and organized. We will later discuss this topic and how it is related to the opinion of nurses, but this dividing line between state and market could be identified as one of the major aspects of possible restructuring processes concerning the health care system. Restructuring in those terms would mean a change in the ratio between health care institutions run within the private and public sector respectively.

Notwithstanding possible changes it is obvious from the table below representing the organizational belongingness of the nurses participating in the study that the absolute major part of the health-care systems are publicly organized, whether by government as in Ireland or by municipalities as in Sweden and Finland.

Table 1. Kind of organization or business in which nurses are employed?

	Governmental / tax financed (%)	Municipality / county council (%)	Profit making companies (%)	Non-profit organisations (%)	Self employed (%)
Finland	5	83	8	3	0,1
Ireland	81	0	12	6	0,7
Sweden	3	86	10	1	0,3

"Q22" refers to question 22 in the English questionnaire (See Sohlberg et al. 2007). In the tables below we will continue to refer to this questionnaire.

This situation with a public responsibility for the institutions of health-care does not conclusively falsify the possibility of a major restructuring on the system level. It could certainly be the case as with New Public Management that the principle of steering, control and accountability are copied from the market and applied within the public sector and thus making market principles rather universal. Another principal possibility concerning restructuring processes in this more general sense is that there could be a change in the relationship between the system- and life-world. In this context this is generally expressed by the metaphor of the system-world as colonizing the life-world, i.e. that power and market-mechanisms are superseding the communicative argumentation of the life-world, or even more concretely put: a loss of power in the everyday work-life.

If we should ourselves apply this communicative rationality when it comes to the balance between market and state, we ought to ask the nurses themselves about their preferences. We have on this subject replicated questions asked in the Wright-studies[12]. where the respondents were asked by what kind of organisation various institutions should be run. The result was the following:

Table 2. How hospitals should be run?

	Finnish nurses (%)	Irish nurses (%)	Swedish nurses (%)
By government/municipality	42	34	41
By government and private companies	57	59	57
By private companies	0,5	7	2

There is only a very small minority of the nurses that prefer hospitals to be uniformly run by private companies and the main preference in all countries is for a mixed model with as well private as public hospitals. This differs somewhat for the analogous situation of the teachers where a rather substantial majority of the teachers prefer secondary schools to be publicly run.[13]

[12] See Wright 1997, 1994.

[13] Swedish teachers are however deviating from this pattern.

Instruments of Governance: Goals and Steering Mechanisms

The general goal-setting and legislation for the health care system is done at a central political and administrative level and it is furthermore generally done by other professionals than nurses. The health-care system and its design is regarded as a legitimate arena for varying political opinions and resulting conflicts regardless of the position (should this even be unitary) of the professions involved in its daily practice. This makes at the outset the communicative rationality of Habermas highly marginalized.

In the case that there is only a one-way steering from state or market as described here Habermas would subsume this under the general tendency of the system-worlds colonisation of the life-world (Habermas 1989) Habermas discusses this aspects not explicitly in terms of steering but in terms of integrative mechanisms, i.e. the state is closely related to the integration mechanism of political power whereas the alternative aspect of the system-world – the market – functions in terms of market principles (ibid.). The normative alternative – dialogue by reason – is the integrative principle of the life-world and is also closely related to the ideal-typical representation of a profession. A relative high autonomy has been a traditional criterion of a profession, and this implies a high degree of control of the goals in the work-situation. This cannot be regarded as a constant situation and there are strong indicators that the situation even for the traditional professions, e.g. in the academia, have undergone a radical change in terms of lessened autonomy and self-control (Jary 2002).

The main explicit goals of institutions within the health-care system are decided by politicians, but the executive control of goal-fulfilment in general is exercised by special authorities within the health-care system but under political control. As mainly publicly financed institutions health care institutions have limited control over the choice of patients. A characteristic of the modern welfare state is the citizens' right to health-care and to the same extent health care is a universal right, all patients, with some restrictions, have to be accepted by the system in its totality.[14] The principle of universality is highly correlated with the general legitimacy of the health-care system, which in its turn is important for its financial resources.

The openness of the system with various external agents and mechanisms implies high requirements of adaptability. This requirement is further accentuated by the fact that the health-care system as mentioned often is a matter of political conflicts and new political majorities can initiate reforms. The situation for the nurses within the health-care system is not merely a pressure from several agents but the position as described as a localisation between state and citizen also means an intermediate position between the demands from above and the needs of the patients as met in the daily interaction. This is a position homologous with the "street level" bureaucrat, with the difference that the tasks of the nurses not solely are administrative in relation to the patients (Lipsky 1980).

[14] Privately run health-care institutions are of course exceptions to this principle of universal accessibility.

In the PROFKNOW project we have been discussing new forms of goal-setting and steering-mechanisms inspired by New Public Management, often characterized by indirect steering by financial resources and more specified control-instances. In the terminology of David Jary, when he speaks of professional control, this could be expressed as a transition from a traditional self regulation of a profession with "Trust in paternalistic, self-regulating professional provider organizations" (Jary, 2002, 48) to a mode of ""Expert" external audit" (ibid.). Regardless of whether nurses should be regarded as profession or semi-profession this development is relevant but the direction is in this aspect certainly in direction of a de-professionalisation. This said against the background that professions typically are characterized by the high impact of communicative action within the group, i.e. a high degree of autonomy.

The general development, portrayed in the project with strong tendencies of an amalgamation between the state and the market also complicates the simple categorization of the system-world, but makes the distinction between life-world and system-world not less relevant.

We have so far been discussing the actual forms or mechanisms of goal-setting within the health-care system at the most general level. What about the actual outcome of those processes in the concrete work-setting? From an empirical point of view it is highly questionable to assume that all goals implemented are executed in a mechanical and uncomplicated way without being "moulded" by the organisational settings and by those responsible for the actual contact with patients. These are practices developed in the social field.

THE SOCIAL FIELD OF HEALTH-CARE

The social field according to Bourdieu is a delimited social arena with hierarchical structure with a struggle about positions and the setting where characteristics are evaluated and constructed as symbolic capital (see e.g. Bourdieu 1984).

Important characteristics of the social field of health-care are that there are few hierarchical levels with few opportunities of promotion and a low degree of autonomy. During the last decades there has been an upgrading of the relative position of this field as the education of nurses has been integrated within the university system.

In contrast with the teachers the social field of health-care is characterized by a more complex hierarchy relevant for the everyday work, including several occupations such as nurses' assistants and doctors. There is furthermore no possibility of upgrading or promotion between those categories within the field but such a career necessitates an upgrading within the educational system. Nurses also have a mandatory authorization as a requirement for fulfilling their position in contrast with teachers e.g. in Sweden. At the level of work-place nurses' work is embedded in a much more hierarchical setting than what applies for teachers. Nurses are generally positioned in an intermediary level where doctors have more power whereas teachers in general work together with colleagues.

Decisions about what constitutes symbolic capital are primarily made outside the field and not decided primarily through struggles within the field even though there are minor differentiations of symbolic capital within the occupation. We thus have a situation where forces in the system-world set many of the standards and rules of the social field of health-care.

There is however a difference between the fields of health-care and education in the sense that most patients only have a rather short contact with the health-care system whereas pupils in the school have a continuous contact with the educational system for many years. [15] In terms of Parsons pattern-variables one can express this as concerning the dimension diffuseness–specificity, where the role of the health care system in its totality is more specified and closely defined than that of the educational system (Parsons & Shils 1951). There is however an interesting similarity between the educational and the health-care system in that debate on health care and education often are initiated by mass media and have great impact as a bearer of political conflicts and divergences of interests. Furthermore important in this digitalized world nurses as well as teachers produce services for the local market and their particular service provided binds producers and consumers to the same locale (see Giddens 1984).

Possible restructuring when related to developments in the social fields of health care could have to do with changes of the hierarchical structure e.g. number of positions and career trajectories; the substance of symbolic capital such as the relative value of experience based skills vs. formal education in specific subjects. A major change of this field has been the academisation of nurses' education where there this development has opened up for career opportunities within the universities. It is however an open question as to the degree to which this has affected the actual field relevant for practising nurses or if it has been an alternative academic labour market.

A difference between the social field of health-care and the educational system is that the health-care system does not have a corresponding hierarchy as the educational system, based on different levels of the clients, i.e. primary, secondary and tertiary education with a homologous hierarchy of teachers. It is not self-evident that a differentiation between e.g. specialized nurses working at university hospitals and nurses working in primary care corresponds to the distinctions within the social field of education with corresponding effects on wages and status. When studying the hierarchical structure of the social field matters of control and supervision are crucial.

Promotion, Supervision and Control

Supervision and control could be viewed from two positions in this work-life setting, i.e. to be subject of supervision and control and to exercise supervision and control over others

[15] That this contact with the health-care system is rather sporadic is e.g. reflected in the decrease of number of hospital beds during the last decades.

In the survey we asked the question: "*My work is more controlled and supervised nowadays*" in order to capture the general and subjective experience of control. We found here, in contrast with the situation for teachers, rather small differences between nurses from different countries, where 53% of the Irish nurses and 62% of the Swedish nurses agreed with this statement.[16] A majority of the nurses (87-69 percent) answered that their supervisors check their work less than once a week. The Irish nurses are more often controlled than Finnish and Swedish nurses.

Direct control occurs rather seldom, which can be interpreted as supervisors' trust of the nurses' professionalism. The implication is also that the positive aspect of supervision e.g. talking about competence development also occurs rather seldom. About two of five Swedish and almost the same ratio of Finnish nurses say that they regularly talk about competence development, compared with one of five Irish nurses.

The statement of more "control" and "supervision" is easily interpreted as a normative statement with negative content, but this interpretation is not self-evident. Only app. 1/3 of the nurses agreed with the statement that "*The non-management employees in my place of work could run things effectively without bosses*", which seem to imply some acceptance of the control of supervisors.

Even if a big part of nurses perceive an increase of supervision and control they do not at the concrete level experience that they personally are controlled very often. More than two of three of them are not controlled as often as once a week.[17]

The fact that nurses state that they seldom are controlled in an explicit and apparent way shifts the focus to other forms of control of a more indirect kind. An important possible explanation of the fact that majority the nurses do not experience control from supervisors as an influential factor in their daily work is that they understand "control" in a narrow way, as direct regulation of their actions from supervisors. This form of control is probably rather unusual towards professionally educated employees. Control of these groups mostly occurs indirectly in more complex forms of steering, when e.g. supervisor exercises "ideological" influence, put resources to disposal for someone or evaluate his or hers job. In that broader sense, control is merged with leadership and can even in the best of worlds include tutorial and advice.

We then have the other aspect of supervision – being in a supervisory position. This is also related to the active aspect of the professional habitus.

In contrast with the teachers where only one of four have a supervisory position more than 60% of the nurses have a supervisory position, reflecting that they are part of a hierarchical structure with subordinate positions. This situation is most pronounced in Ireland where almost 80 % of the nurses state that they supervise work of others.

The system of supervision is one side of the organisational structure, describing relations of control between individuals in the organisation. The system of promotion

---

[16] Among teachers on the contrary there are big differences between the national cases concerning this statement.

[17] The percentages of nurses stating that they are controlled once a week or more often are for the Irish nurses 30 percent and for the Finnish and Swedish nurses, between 17 and 12 percent respectively.

describes another aspect of the organisational structure, namely the individuals' chances to reach higher position in organisation step by step.[18]

The frequency of promotions depends on how the occupation is hierarchically structured. The finer the gradation of positions the bigger chance to get promotion. The survey shows as a general tendency that nurses not have been promoted to any appreciable extent and only a minority of them have been promoted several times.

Table 3. Were you ever promoted?

	Promoted several times (%)	Promoted once (%)	Never (%)	Total
Finland	6	24	70	779
Ireland	17	29	54	621
Sweden	15	20	64	783

Dependency Coefficient between nurses from different countries is 0.167 significant at 0.00 level.

The organisation of nurses' job does not consist of a steady hierarchic upgrading. However there are some differences between countries where Irish nurses are promoted to a higher degree than the Finnish and Swedish nurses. Seen from a professional perspective it is remarkable that such a great part of the Finnish and Swedish nurses never have been promoted.

It is thus rather obvious that there are not any clear career trajectories for nurses in their original work-setting, i.e. that their "internal" social field is characterized by a formal hierarchy with few positions. This also implies that the possible continuous upgrading of skills and knowledge is of minor importance in a career perspective.

Many of the items concerned with power and control, so far discussed and even more to come is a matter of subjective estimates and general attitudes. We consider them crucial for understanding the every-day work of nurses in accordance with the Thomas-theorem that emphasizes the individual's interpretation of situations for her actions (Thomas 1928). The acceptance of this does not however exclude the importance of the factual and constraining conditions existing in the organisation where teachers and nurses work. To those factual conditions we regard the influence over major decisions affecting the organisation of the work-place. We will later return to this interface between life- and system-world.

Restructuring is of course a dynamic concept referring to changes over time. The survey technique covers principally only static pictures, but in order to capture possible aspects of restructuring we asked retrospective questions about developments of the social field and the work-situation in general. The respondents were asked to respond to various statements concerning their work and work-situation:

[18] The interesting paradox would be if – in light of the discourse or the rhetoric of life long-learning – there would be no trajectories of promotion in the organisation. There would then be no obvious correspondence between the requests on the individual and the opportunities provided by the organisation.

Table 4. When you look back to the day when you started to work in your occupation as a nurse – What are your general impressions today, compared with earlier? Percentage agreeing (strongly or somewhat).

	Finnish nurses Agree	Irish nurses Agree	Swedish nurses Agree	Contingency coefficient Finnish-Irish	Contingency coefficient Finnish-Swedish	Contingency coefficient Irish-Swedish
Demand of written documentation increased	92	97	93	0.220	(0.048)	0.188
The work climate has become more demanding	92	95	88	0.145	0.193	0.307
More team-work nowadays	79	74	70	0.097*	0.257	0.209
Spending more time explaining work to others	63	88	54	0.301	0.207	0.399
More competition between hospitals	53	61	60	(0.090)	0.154	0.118
My work is more controlled	57	54	62	(0.041)	0.095	0.133
Nurses have achieved more authority	52	76	46	0.257	0.127	0.346
Less of hierarchies nowadays	54	38	62	0.245	0.120	0.337
Work is more routinised nowadays	32	51	44	0.230	0.224	0.205
My professional expertise is more questioned	29	83	34	0.491	0.205	0.480
My education was more appreciated earlier	35	53	28	0.179	0.139	0.280

* Significant at 0.01 level; in parenthesis – not significant at 0.01 level, all other significant at 0.00 level. Coefficients are counted on all values except "cannot decide." The share of those who answered "cannot decide" varied from 2 percent to 15 (The highest value is for "more competition").

The differences between Finland/Sweden and Ireland concerning attitudes about changes in work condition are in most cases very strong whereas the differences between the Nordic countries are minor. Relating the two occupations in our study there is a very important difference between nurses and teachers concerning the perception of changes in authority. A great part of the nurses agreed with that statement of increased authority but only about 10 percent of the teachers agreed with this statement.

The social field of nursing as well as the social field of education seem to have become somewhat more conflict-loaded, with harder demands as well from external forces (more competition and documentation), and from the inside (more team-work and an increased demand of explaining work to others). For the teachers this situation happens together with a perception of a lessened authority of the occupation whereas this negative perception not is as apparent for the nurses.

All opinions described above capture general tendencies as nurses regard them. It is not necessarily so that they constitute concrete changes in the individuals' concrete work-setting. They can express the ideological climate, and mirror general discourses about changes.

Even though the social field of health-care has a low degree of autonomy and is in the middle of counteracting forces this and adjacent fields are anyhow the relevant context for understanding the construction of symbolic capital. What characterizes the processes of evaluation and what kind of characteristics are emphasized in this process?

The Symbolic Capital in the Field of Health Care

When discussing the status of a given profession the principal view could be regarded as a matter of market position, organizational strength and power of "consecration" (Bourdieu 1984; Weber 1978). Only to focus on organizational strength and the ability to closure would be too limited and the symbolic value of the professional knowledge also has to be taken into consideration.

It should be stressed that the categorization in terms of profession, professional knowledge etc. not should be a normative decision from the social scientists point of view. By characterizing knowledge as professional or an occupation as a profession the idea is rather to depict the actual valuations done in the social fields by agents with power to establish symbolic capital. Professional knowledge could be analyzed from various perspectives concerning the hierarcisation of professional fields. It could concern the professional habitus from various aspects, e.g. the opportunities to update knowledge by participating on conferences, attend courses etc. An absolute dividing criterion in this aspect is *not* passive forms of upgrading and collecting information relevant for the field in question, but the opportunity to actually participate in the production of knowledge. As we will see below it is extremely seldom that nurses, working in the health care sector spend time on research or other kind of systematic knowledge-production relevant for their work.

In old academic theories of stratification (e.g. Davis & Moore 1945) as well as in many modern discourses of stratification and professional status (Grusky 2008; Scott 1996), a fundamental explanatory variable of income-inequalities and status-hierarchies has to do with the ability of a professional group to have some degree of monopoly of valuable characteristics. This could thus be expressed in terms of properties necessary, though scarce, for the maintenance of the social system (Davis & Moore 1945), social closure (Weber 1978), or control of the establishment of symbolic capital in the social field (Bourdieu 1984, 1992)

Somewhat superficially this could be summarized as some kind of market-power of the professional group in question. This market-power in its turn has to do with the ability of the professional group to control the "supply-side" of the profession in question. Another aspect of the market power of the profession, beside the aspect of scarcity that was highlighted in the above referred article by Davis and Moore is the functional importance of the properties in question assumed to be part of the profession.

An interesting aspect of those crucial characteristics, i.e. symbolic capital in Bourdieu's terms is their general legitimacy in a wider context than the specific field. When introducing the conception of symbolic capital Bourdieu emphasizes social and power-aspects of values, i.e. the valuation of characteristics is seen as the outcome of a social process involving social conflicts and in the context of a hierarchy. Symbolic capital as concept is characterized by its plasticity and its systematic social character involving also conflicts on the social field where it is constituted. The plasticity has to do with an empirical openness for what characteristics are actually evaluated and rewarded at the specific social field in question.

If we now apply the aspect of consecration, or power to form and evaluate symbolic capital, we find that nurses have an interesting and changing relation vis-à-vis academia. The parallel relation between the occupation and academia has also changed for the teachers but in a somewhat different way. As the education for nurses to a high degree have been integrated within the university system e.g. in forms of caring science, new career opportunities have developed for nurses. At least in the long run one could expect some feedback of this research for the practical work as a nurse, but seen in its totality the knowledge-production done within traditional medical research is dominant and thus characterizing the hierarchy within the field.

What is then the nurses own conception of how their education is appreciated? We asked this question in the retrospective fashion mentioned above.

Table 5. My education was more appreciated in the beginning of my working career divided by working time.

	Finnish nurses (%)	Irish nurses (%)	Swedish nurses (%)
Working 1-10 years	25	51	14
Working 11-25 years	39	49	28
Working more than 25 years	43	62	41
Kendall's tau b	0.126	(0.062)	0.243

Only responses agreeing with the statement are presented here (alternatives: agree somewhat and strongly). Correlations are of course estimates of all values except "cannot decide".

As we can see the differences between countries are rather big with somewhat of a dividing line between the Nordic countries and Ireland. In contrast with the Finnish and Swedish nurses, the majority of the Irish nurses are convinced that their professional education was more appreciated earlier.

It is also remarkable that even the relatively new-graduated nurses to such a high degree say that their education was more appreciated earlier. A reasonable understanding of this is that they to some extent are evaluating the conception of the occupation as such and not only evaluating their own occupational career.

The diachronic aspect of how education is appreciated must be seen partly in context of the increasing number of people with tertiary education, partly in context of their own parents' education

Nurses Formal Education and Material Rewards

The professional education of nurses is rather heterogeneous what concerns its position within the educational system. There are still a big part of them who have secondary school or college as their highest education, while a part of them have education at university level. Comparing with teachers, there is a smaller part of the nurses that have university education.

Table 6. Highest educational level of nurses presented by country.

	Secondary school or college (%)	Bachelor or similar education (%)	M.A. or similar (%)	Other (%)
Finnish nurses	76	21	1	2
Irish nurses	43	43	4	9
Swedish nurses	37	42	9	12

Non-university educations are placed in the category secondary school or college. This could give the impression that Finnish nurses have a less qualified education than what is the case. Finnish nurses have since 1987 had a matriculation exam of 3, 5 years.

There are differences between countries and generations concerning educational content and level, which differences reflects variation in the structural conditions and changes in the educational systems which have occurred during the last forty years. Table 6 above represents a static picture of the educational level summarizing the formal educational capital of the nurses. An interesting aspect of the educational system is also the dynamic aspect, e.g. not to focus only on the educational level at the entrance of the working life as nurse, but to capture the possibility of educational upgrading as well as education attended before the training as a nurse.

Figure 1. Educational dynamics. When nurses received their additional education in relation to the nurse education. The minimum length of this additional education here presented is half a year (%).

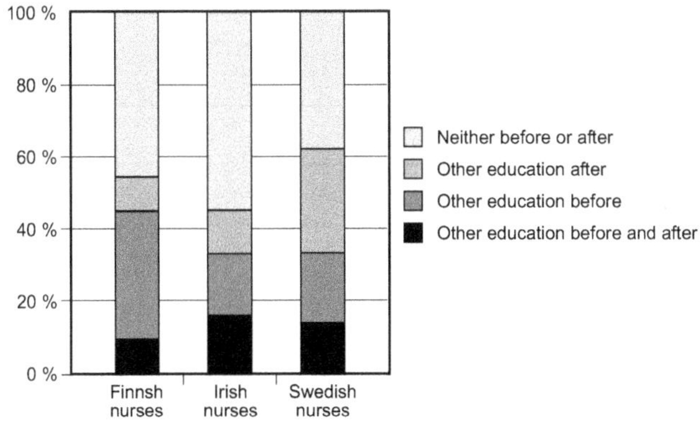

The general picture is that most nurses neither have a professional education before the training as a nurse nor any additional education after graduation. We can see that there are clear differences between Sweden and Finland where many Swedish nurses have additional education after their basic education. If we study the "extreme" group (those with no additional education neither before nor after their education as nurses), we find that this group is rather small compared with the corresponding figure for teachers, with some exception for the Swedish nurses. Seen in the context of professionalism and knowledge-society the need of updating knowledge has to be considered. If the mean working time of nurses in our sample is 16 years the implication is that there has not been a possibility of upgrading the knowledge within the traditional academic system for quite a while.

The main material reward in the social field of education is the wage. The wage system reveals a lot of information about the social field of an occupation e.g. to what extent meritocratic qualities are emphasized; if we have to deal with formal bureaucratic principles, or if there is room for informal or even nepotistic relations. The system of wage-setting also gives a picture of power-relations and how powerful the employees are in negotiations with employers.

The respondents were asked about to what extent possible factors could influence people's pay rates at their work-place.[19]

The result in an aggregated form could be described as some kind of fusion between different national wage-systems and specific circumstances relevant for the work-place in question. The question is phrased in order for respondents to give a general estimate of principles relevant for their work-place in general.

Table 7. Factors which influence pay rise.

	Finnish nurses (%)	Irish nurses (%)	Swedish nurses (%)	Tau-b Finland -Ireland	Tau-b Finland -Sweden	Tau-b Ireland - Sweden
Good work				0.180	0.537	0.579
Definitely + probably true	14	13	63			
Probably + definitely false	77	84	27			
Don't know	10	3	10			
How long working				0.205	0.238	(0.060)
Definitely + probably true	24	53	40			
Probably + definitely false	68	45	47			
Don't know	7	2	12			
More education or training				(0.008)	0.510	0.403
Definitely + probably true	22	34	71			
Probably + definitely false	71	63	20			
Don't know	7	4	9			
Close connections with important people				0.111	0.308	0.385
Definitely + probably true	12	11	26			
Probably + definitely false	84	83	61			
Don't know	4	5	13			
Formal position				0.277	0.236	0.473
Definitely + probably true	55	75	27			
Probably + definitely false	37	17	57			
Don't know	8	8	17			

Coefficients are calculated on all values except "don't know". In parentheses – correlations are not significant at 0.01 level.

[19] These questions are replicated from the Wright-studies (see Wright 1997).

The Finnish and Irish nurses state that good work does not influence pay rise whereas a majority of the Swedish nurses, interesting from a perspective of motivation, is of another opinion. The differences are in many cases stronger between Sweden and the other countries than between the Nordic countries and Ireland. Swedish nurses, in contrast to Irish and Finnish nurses, regard not formal position to be a crucial factor for pay rise. The majority of the nurses do not regard close connections with important people as a significant factor for pay rise. Important from the profession perspective is the relatively low importance of more education for pay rise.

The phrasing of the question strongly imply that the picture obtained is not merely a subjective attitudinal matter but rather a perception of an actual situation. The principal situation can be summed up as follow: if formal position is the most important factor for pay rise we probably have a formal bureaucratic organisation in a Weberian sense where there are predefined steps in a hierarchical trajectory and where time spent in the organisation probably, but not necessarily, is the crucial factor. Stress on educational efforts is characteristic of a meritocracy and also connected to the received view of professionalism. The implication of systems rewarding good work depends on how transparent and by which criteria this is judged. It could be more or less being based on nepotism. A de-centralized, non-formalized system and accordingly non-transparent system in general makes personal relations more important.

So far our main focus has been on describing the theoretical context of nurses' every-day activities on the most general systemic level and on the intermediate level in terms of social fields. It is now time to centre more on the actual activities, perceptions and attitudes.

Where the Life World Meets the System-world

A main theme of the PROFKNOW project has been work-life under systematic change or transition. As a holistic indicator of the experiences of restructuring processes we asked the respondents of their experience of organisational changes, i.e. if they have experienced a lot of organisational changes.

Table 8. I have experienced a lot of organisational changes (%).

	Generation			Correlation with generation
	Working as a nurse -10 years	Working as a nurse 11-25 years	Working as a nurse more than 25 years	Kendall's tau b
Finland	39	62	67	0.245
Ireland	84	89	98	0.216
Sweden	71	89	95	0.281

Percentage of all who have answered "very true" or "quite true."

The experience of changes increase rapidly with increased time spent in working within the occupation for the Finnish nurses. The majority of the Irish and Swedish nurses, even those who have been working a relative short time, have experienced a lot of organisational changes.

It is hardly surprising that the experience of organisational changes is escalating with increasing time in work-life. The statement responded to is in itself normatively neutral. Organizational changes could theoretically imply improvements as well as deterioration. In our other findings concerning changes in more concrete work-tasks does however indicate that those changes not are experienced as improvements. For the static picture of nurses' work-life practice we have a detailed picture of actual tasks as well as influencing factors and obstacles.

What are then nurses actually doing when working? In the diagram below we find a distribution of the main activities:

Figure 2. Nurses main duties (%).

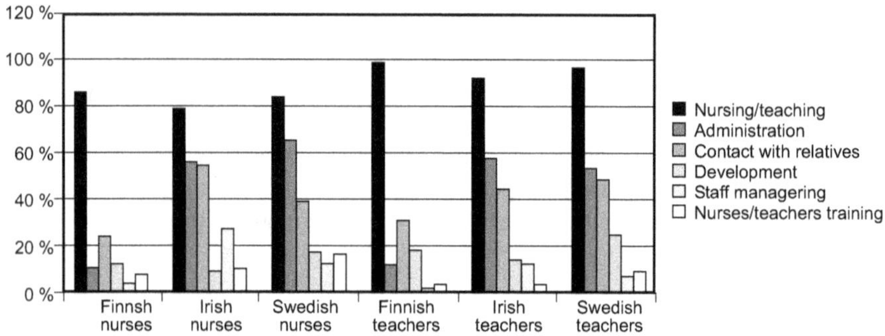

It is obvious that what could be called the basic activities i.e. nursing dominate the work-day. Furthermore administration and contact with relatives take a great part of the time for both occupations, with the exception of Finnish nurses. What is interesting in the perspective of traditional profession is that only a small proportion of the work-time is spent with research activities.[20] The same applies to trade-union activities.[21]

The idea of a common Nordic model is contested by this distribution of activities. Finnish nurses are e.g. highly professional in a traditional way, i.e. they concentrate on the main activity i.e. nursing and spend very little time on administration and

[20] The same could be said of traditional professions as e.g. doctors, architects and lawyers. The difference is however that for these professions there is no "competing" occupation in the university systems producing knowledge that should be applied in their practice. For teachers those competing occupations integrated in the university system is (academics within the specialist subjects (the cognitive dimension) and pedagogues (practical skills)).

[21] Those activities are so marginal that they not are included in the diagram.

other side-activities.

In order to capture not only the concrete activities but also the context of those, we asked the nurses about factors influencing their work:

Table 9. How much do the following factors influence your daily work (%)?

	Finnish nurses	Irish nurses	Swedish nurses
Own conception of work	94	91	90
Opinion of patients	76	74	79
Demand of documentation	78	81	84
Planning with colleagues	65	65	71
Evaluation of work	45	53	30
The risk of being sued	41	54	31
Control of supervisors	24	29	25
Mass media coverage	12	29	13
Competition with other hospitals	9	10	13

Percentages of those who answered "very much" and ""rather much"

As we can see, the general opinion of changes described above in table 4 and the static perspective about factors influencing daily work are not fully convergent. Even though a great majority stated that the work-climate has become more demanding, we can here see that an even bigger majority find their own conception of work as highly influential for their daily work.

Unlike teachers for whom the opinion of pupils and planning with colleagues next after own conception of work were the most important factors influencing their daily work, the demand of documentation is highlighted as a main factor for nurses. The risk of being sued, although it is not as important as own conception and or demand of documentation, is clearly more important for nurses than for teachers as also is control from supervisors. Nurses' daily work is more monitored by others than teachers work, at least according to the respondent themselves.

What then about the actual substance of the obstacles for the unexpectedly small group experiencing them? When asking this we found the following pattern[22]:

[22] In this table we have included those experiencing serious obstacles several times per month. Percentage of those who agreed with the statement of this restricted group.

Table 10. Serious obstacles for carrying through own ideas coming from (%).

	Finnish nurses	Irish nurses	Swedish nurses
Lack of time	31	44	18
Lack of economic resources	16	43	17
Work organisation	26	36	17
Legislation and steering documents	15	34	9
Supervisors	21	27	14
Computer equipment	17	30	9
Lack of professional training	12	23	2
My colleagues	12	20	7
Patients relatives	9	20	1
Patients	6	13	1

There are rather big differences between countries in this respect: The Irish nurses differ from as well the Finnish and the Swedish nurses as more of the Irish nurses experience serious obstacles. There are however some differences between the Finnish and Swedish nurses, e.g. fewer of the Swedish nurses experience lack of time and lack of professional training as serious obstacles than the Finnish nurses.

A test of the degree of the system-world's colonisation of the life-world would in this context be the control of various aspects of the work-situation externally influencing the work-situation, primarily aspects related to active decision making.

CONTROL, PARTICIPATION AND DECISION

It has become rather a fashion to use Foucault in various fields to illustrate diverse forms of oppressive forms of control-mechanisms as an essential part of social life and more general to identify a general trajectory from external control to self-discipline.[23]

A problem with the mechanical application of the Foucaldian notion of control on our data has to do with the focus on manifest aspects of control and its problematic implementation in complex organizational settings. How e.g. to interpret the relationship between different levels of control? Below we will contrast the rather positive picture of nurses and teachers influence over their working day with more structural aspects, where the idea of self-control seems far-fetched, and where it is more plausible to use the conventional conception of a structural domination where power actually has a specific locus

Less principal, but not less important, problems in this context with applying a priori a notion of self-repressive control to our findings has to do with an aspect that Giddens has called the duality of structure. Giddens phrasing of this idea is,

[23] Related to Foucault's reluctance to universal theories and the post-modern tradition's emphasis on local knowledge it's somewhat surprising that these general schemes have become so widespread.

if we focus on the programmatic aspect, that the structure sets limitations as well as provides resources for action (Giddens 1984, 25ff). How could we at all assume the possibility of resistance-strategies, resulting in refractions of structural changes, if we do not accept the possibility of nurses not only subordinating to structural changes, but actually acting on basis of their professional competence in spite of those changes, should they be contradictory to their interests? On the other hand, it would be utterly unrealistic to consider the restructuring processes as the sole outcome of nurses' actions in their everyday working life.

Applying the programmatic notion of duality of structure to our concrete material we thus have to take into consideration structural aspects as well as resources as limitations and restrictions. In the survey we have several items covering different aspects of control-mechanisms, i.e. supervision, requirements of documentation and we have seen that the nurses find that they are not to a high degree hindered to realize their own ideas in the work-place setting. What about more strategic decisions concerning their work-place?

The Influence over Strategic Decisions

In what way can nurses influence allocations of resources within the work-place and the services delivered by the organisation? We have here crucial factors setting the more long-term conditions of work-practice. When asking about varying degrees of influence over strategic decisions, we found the following:

Table 11. Participation in policy decision (%).

	Finnish nurses	Irish nurses	Swedish nurses
Decisions about distribution of funds			
Participate directly	6	8	6
Give advice	22	13	9
Decisions about increasing or decreasing of personal			
Participate directly	3	6	5
Give advice	30	13	14
Decisions about changes in method of work			
Participate directly	26	21	24
Give advice	50	37	53
Decisions about services delivered by organisation			
Participate directly	6	39	10
Give advice	22	0	27

Percentage of those who answered. The response "no" (influence) not included

Quite a big ratio of all nurses do *not* participate in decisions concerning the distribution of funds, decreasing or increasing of personal and about services delivered by organisation in which they work. Differences between countries are small. The only decisions which nurses have some influence over are changes in method of work.

Seen in contrast with our earlier discussion about a great proportion of nurses not feeling any serious obstacles in realizing their ideas, and the absence of external control etc., those figures are really dramatic in the contrasting picture they show. We can also here discern the importance of studying aspects of power and control at different levels. If we instead study the complimentary situation of non-control we would have an operationalisation of powerlessness concerning vital aspects of the work situation:

Table 12. Powerlessness: respondents who neither participate directly in decision nor give advice. Generation and educational level (%).

	Generation			Education	
	Working as a nurse -10 years	Working as a nurses 11-25 years	Working as a nurses more than 25 years	College or similar	University
Finland	57	45	48	49	54
Ireland	55	51	49	55	50
Sweden	69	53	51	53	60

Percentage of all who have answered"no" on questions 39-1, 39-2 and 39-4.

There are thus rather small differences between nurses with various working length strongly indicating that the small influence over strategic decisions is not a problem for those in the beginning of the career, with some exception for the Swedish nurses. We can also see that formal education is not a crucial factor influencing power over strategic decisions.

When discussing power one should distinguish between power mainly emanating from individuals (e.g. supervision) and directed mostly at the concrete individual on the one hand and more structural aspects on the other hand that is in effect continually during the working day. When we are talking about the kind of decisions mentioned above – we change focus, because these decisions influence simultaneously many individuals working on the same working place and those decisions are in general made a few times per year, and with really long-lasting consequences. In this case power seems to be de-personalized in Foucaldian sense. If we step up one level in the organizational hierarchy we find that further decisions are made setting the limitations of the decisions at the concrete work-place.

As can be seen in the table there are relatively few nurses with substantial influence on decisions concerning their own work-place.

DISCUSSION

In a meritocratic society one of the few principles with some legitimacy for the hierarchical ordering and uneven distribution of resources and rewards is differences in education. Traditional professions have often gained their position and status via the educational system originally in a time where university education was reserved for the elite. Knowledge acquired in the formal educational system seems then to be a crucial factor. However, in the discourses about knowledge, knowledge-society and knowledge related to professionalism, the actual content and substance of knowledge is seldom discussed. Knowledge tends to be approached in a roundabout procedural way and given some general and rather diffuse properties e.g. as being constantly in flux and in need of updating etc.

It could be argued that discourses concerning occupations emanating from the idea of a vocation and where women early made an entrance on the labour-market, to a high degree are focused on personal and moral characteristics of the possessor and a strong polarization between cognitive and practical skills.

Regardless of how we operationalise the concept of profession and study the development of diverse occupational groups according to some professionalisation-scale, we miss one fundamental aspect of the relation between life- and system-world, i.e. what could be called the professional capacity of the labour market. If we instead focus on the labour-market in general we could focus on its properties concerning professionalisation, i.e. the capacity of the labour market to absorb professional qualities of the work-force. A criterion for judging this would be if there are systematically developed receptors sensible for the professional standards of the occupations and if there is a reciprocal communication between the professions and the policy-makers. There is however strong evidence in our findings that point in the opposite direction, i.e. that the demand of formal qualifications have increased, but the actual impact and influence on basis of professional knowledge has decreased, i.e. a lack of professional capacity of the labour-market.

CONCLUSIONS IN A CROSS-PROFESSIONAL PERSPECTIVE:

As well nurses as teachers have a rather strong position on the labour market, but there is a great discrepancy between the occupations in that nurses to a higher degree have a positive expectation to get an alternative job.

There is a great discrepancy between the holistic subjective experience of control of the work-situation and the actual influence on substantial decisions influencing the everyday-work.

There is a great discrepancy between nurses and teachers concerning their estimate of the authority of their own profession when the nurses have a much more positive conception.

The social field of nursing and teaching have an organizational structure with few promotions and career-trajectories and the working teachers and nurses are only to a low degree involved in the systematic knowledge-production relevant for their field.

The "Scandinavian model" of nursing and health-care seems to be as heterogeneous concerning professional education and work-tasks of nurses and teachers, as to make it reasonable to question it as a unitary model.

In light of the low possibilities of promotion and few systematic opportunities to update the knowledge one can question the professional capacity of the labour-market of nurses and teachers.

REFERENCES

Ahrne, G. & Papakostas, A. (2002). *Organisationer, samhälle och globalisering. Tröghetens mekanismer och förnyelsens förutsättningar*. Lund: Studentlitteratur.

Archer, M. (2003). *Structure, Agency and the Internal Conversation*. Cambridge: Cambridge University Press.

Beach, D. (Ed.) (2005). *Welfare State Restructuring in Education and Health Care: Implications for the Teaching and Nursing Professions and their Professional Knowledge*. Report No. 2 from the PROFKNOW- project. http://www.profknow.net/files/results/WP2.pdf

Bourdieu, P. (1984). *Distinction. A Social Critique of the Judgement of Taste*. Cambridge, Massachusetts:Harvard University Press.

Bourdieu P. et al. (1991). *The Craft of Sociology: Epistemological Preliminaries*. Berlin & New York: Walter de Gruyter.

Bourdieu. P. (1992). *The Logic of Practice*. Cambridge & Oxford: Polity Press.

Davis, K. & Moore, W.E. (1945): Some Principles of Stratification. *American Sociological Review*, 10 (2), 242-249.

Giddens. A. (1984). *The Constitution of Society: Outline of the Theory of Structuration*. Cambridge: Polity Press.

Goodson I. & Norrie, C. (2005). *A Literature Review of Welfare State Restructuring in Education and Health Care in European Contexts: Implications for the Teaching and Nursing Professions and their Professional Knowledge*. Report No. 1 from the PROFKNOW- project. www.Profknow.net.

Grusky, D.B. (Ed.) (2008). *Social Stratification. Class, Race and Gender in Sociological Perspective*. Colorado: Westview Press.

Habermas, J. (1989). *The Theory of Communicative Action. Volume 2. Lifeworld and System: A Critique of Functionalist Reason*. Cambridge, Oxford: Polity Press.

Jary, D. (2002). *Aspects of the "Audit Society": issues arising from colonization of professional academic identities by a "portable management tool". In M. Dent & S. Whitehead. 2002. Knowledge, Performativity and the "New" Professional*. London; Routledge Studies in Business Organizations and Networks, Routledge.

Kosonen, T. & Houtsonen J. (Eds.) (2007). *European Nurses' Life and Work under Restructuring: Professional Experiences, Knowledge and Expertise in Changing Contexts*. Deliverable 5, Profknow-project, www.Profknow.net

Layder. D. (2006). *Understanding Social Theory*. 2. ed. Sage: London.

Leiulfsrud, H. & Sohlberg, P. (1996). Contextualizing Social Stratification in Comparative Research in R. Blom et al. *Between Plan and Market. Social Change in the Baltic States and Russia*. Berlin, New York: Walter de Gruyter.

Lipsky, M. (1980). *Street-level Bureaucracy: Dilemmas of the Individual in Public Services*. New York:Russel Sage Foundation.

Mouzelis. N. (1995). *Sociological Theory: What Went Wrong. Diagnosis and Remedies*. London: Routledge.

Müller, J. Hernández, F. Sancho. J. Creus, A. Muntadas,M. Larrain,V. Giro,X. (Eds.) (2007). *European schoolteachers work and life under restructuring: Professional experiences, knowledge and expertise in changing context*. Deliverable 4 Profknow-project. www.Profknow.net

Nightingale, F. (1969). [1860]. Notes on Nursing. What it is, and What it is Not. New York: Dover Publications.

Parsons, T. & Shils E. (1951). *Toward a General Theory of Action*. New York: Harper & Row.

Ruben, D.H. (Ed.)(1993). *Explanation*. Oxford: Oxford University Press.

Scott, J. (1996). *Stratification & Power. Structures of Class, Status and Command*. Cambridge: Polity Press.

Scott, R. (1998). *Organisations, Rational, Natural and Open Systems*. UK; Prentice-Hall International.

Sohlberg P. Czaplicka, M. Lindblad, S. Houtsonen J. Müller, J. Morgan, M. Wärvik, G-B. Dupont, M. Norris, C. Kitching, K. Kosonen, T. (2007). *Professional Expertise under Restructuring: Comparative Studies of Education and Health Care*: The Survey Study. www.Profknow.net

Thomas, W. I. (1928). *The Child in America. Behaviour Problems and Programs*. New York: Alfred A. Knopf.

Weber. M. (1978). *Economy and Society. An Outline of Interpretative Sociology*. Vol 1 Part Two, Berkeley, Los Angeles, London: University of California Press.

Wright, E.O. (1994). *Interrogating Inequality. Essays on Class Analysis. Socialism and Marxism*. London and New York: Verso.

Wright. E.O. (1997). *Class Counts. Comparative Studies in Class Analysis*. Cambridge; Cambridge University Press.

APPENDIX

The PROFKNOW survey is integrated as one of the tools of data-collection within the project and its rationale is to give an overall comprehensive view of teachers and nurses situation as a supplementary method together with research reviews and qualitative studies (Müller et al. 2007; Kosonen & Houtsonen 2007).

The survey material was collected from nurses and teachers in autumn 2005 and spring 2006. Initial samples were 1,100 nurses and 1,100 teachers in each country. In relation to what is now standard for postal-surveys the response rate must be considered as rather high. Furthermore the respondents do not differ in sex-composition and level of education from the corresponding populations and it may be assumed that this survey gives a good representation of the whole population of nurses and teachers in the countries participating.

The survey covers persons in an age-span of forty years: the youngest nurses and teachers being born 1981 and the oldest being born in 1941.

JARMO HOUTSONEN & TONI KOSONEN

EUROPEAN NURSES ARTICULATING CARE

INTRODUCTION

Previous research (Bassett 2002; Kirpal 2003) and our national case studies (Dupont & Sugrue 2007; Kosonen and Houtsonen 2007a; Kosonen and Houtsonen 2007b; Müller et al. 2007; Norrie & Goodson 2007; Pereira 2007; Safilou-Rothschild 2007; Wärvik 2007) suggest that nurses' professional self-identity is organised around the category of nursing care. In this paper we describe how nurses in the seven European countries studied in the PROFKNOW project articulated nursing care in their interviews. We do not offer an objective definition or complete typology of nursing care, but simply describe nurses' comprehension of their work in various national and local health care settings in an era of restructuring health care in Europe.

What emerges in our analysis of interviews is that nurses tend to offer manifold articulations of nursing care. The idea of care does not seem have any definite core or unambiguous meaning, but is articulated in several ways depending on the social relations and conditions. For instance, in relation to medical doctors nursing care is seen as an almost innate quality of a nurse, centred in personal, emotional and social skills coupled with long-term relations with the patient. Indeed, nurses often want to define patient care in opposition to cure – the home turf of doctors – which is seen as impersonal and technical relation to patients. In reality nurses' work also includes various technical and medical skills and knowledge, for instance, their observation and recording of vital functions. By contrast, in relation to nursing assistants and lay people, care is often defined as based on nursing science, learnable at higher education institutes.

We regard various articulations of nursing care, such as the oppositions between cure and care, technical and personal, or bio-medical and humanistic, as symbolic (Durkheim 1965) and practical (Bourdieu 1990) expressions of the social reality of health care, including the organisation of work. In fact, for instance, the opposition between cure and care is rooted in the concrete division of labour between the nurses and the doctors. However, the definition of nursing care or any other symbolic configuration is continuously negotiated, contested and confirmed or gradually transformed.

Our goal is not to compare countries or nurses occupying different positions in order to create a number of typologies. This task would have been interesting and promising. For instance, we could have expected that highly educated specialised nurses working further away from long-term patient relations in laboratory-like settings would emphasise more strongly the technical and bio-medical aspects of

J. Houtsonen, G.-B. Wärvik (Eds.), European Nurses' Life and Work Under Restructuring pp. 59-75.

nursing. Or, we could have tested the hypothesis that the professionalisation of care rather than feminine-like care has proceeded further in the Nordic Countries than in the Southern European Countries characterised as regimes of Late Female Mobilization (see Arts & Gelissen 2002, 149). However, we simply want to describe here how nursing care is understood in various national and local contexts and how current conditions of cost-cutting and steering shape those definitions.

We agree with Carmel (2005), who criticises the dominant discourse in academic nursing science that nursing is solely focused on patient care and is radically distinct from medicine. In reality nurses also take care of the patient's social context, do similar tasks as the doctors, and perform various administrative duties. Although our informants often tend to reproduce the dominant discourse in their narratives, the ambiguities observed in their ideas indicate that the real context and content of their work differs from the idealised picture of nursing care.

CHANGING ROLES AND FUNCTIONS OF NURSING

Professional and occupational roles, functions and tasks in health care, their boundaries and the distribution of work have been changing all over Europe during the past two decades (Bryant-Lukosius et al. 2004). Nurses have been given new tasks because of changes in the idea of health care such as the introduction of preventive care. They have also been given tasks that previously belonged to doctors. Furthermore, some tasks previously performed by nurses are now allocated to various paramedical and auxiliary occupational groups. Various combinations of multi-professional work teams have been introduced in health care settings. Obviously, there are differences in the pace and extension of these transformations but this is the reality in every country targeted in our research project (Goodson & Norrie 2005; Beech 2005). Following Rantalaiho (2004) we consider a profession such as nursing to be a process-like configuration, its shape modified by the changing social and power relations between the state, regions, municipalities, citizens, firms, civic organisations and professional bodies. There is a constant re-organisation of social relations between different professions, altering the ideas of professional knowledge and identity as well.

The diversification of nursing roles, positions, functions and the organisation of work as well as career paths is well illustrated in the case studies of the countries involved in our study (Goodson & Norrie 2005; Beach 2005). Our research informants represented a great variety of nursing roles and tasks, extending from managerial and administrative personnel to specialist and staff nurses. These nurses, different in age and work-experience, too, worked in various settings, ranging from hospital wards to clinics to health centres. In addition, other new occupational groups, such as assistants and health coaches, have entered the scene contributing to the configuration of professional knowledge in nursing as well (Dahle 2003; Daykin and Clark 2000; Nancarrow and Borthwick 2005). While the category of nurse has become more varied, the idea of care, in various modifications, is still at the core of their professional self-identity.

To see nursing as a dynamic configuration is to focus on a constant re-organisation of social relations between different health care professions, which also keeps professional knowledge, identity and status in flux. For example, the institutional re-definitions of doctors' and nurses' tasks, such as the nurses' potential right in the future to prescribe certain common pharmaceuticals, are not just administrative rationalisations in the context of neo-liberal restructuring that re-organise the division of labour and potentially save some money. These changes can also re-define nurses' knowledge, identity and status in relation to doctors, assistants, and patients. Doctors are likely to first give up the 'simple' and 'inferior' tasks, which, however, may strengthen the self-perception and professional status of nurses within society. This change will not necessarily undermine the relative social distance between doctors and nurses, nor generate symbolic and material rewards to the nurses. Nurses also tend to shift dirty, ordinary and routine tasks to the periphery or outside their professional core tasks, keeping their region of knowledge and identity pure and valuable. The washing and feeding of patients is given to nurses' aides and other service staff. Such allocations of tasks are defined not only at the official institutional level, but they are also negotiated at everyday work settings between various individuals and groups of health care staff. These changes and negotiations can produce ambiguous boundaries. For instance, removal eliminating washing and feeding from their work tasks may strengthen nurses' social status and self-esteem, but at the same time they may feel deprived of important opportunities for knowledge and close relations to patients that the feeding and washing sustain. Since nursing is a dynamic configuration and negotiated order, we are likely to observe ambiguities in nurses' articulations about care.

Our previous reports (Beach 2005; Goodson & Norrie 2005; Kosonen & Houtsonen 2007) show that the above organisational changes, proven by our survey as well (see Sohlberg et al. in this book), are paralleled by a set of adjustments in nursing practice and knowledge across the contexts. That is, nursing practice and knowledge have also become more varied. There was evidence in our national reports of such novelties as teamwork, the multidisciplinary approach, extensive use of ICT, evidence-based practice, nurse's reception, nursing research, prescribing medicine, health education and preventive health care, planning, building up nursing services, administration, management, teaching, and documentation. These broadening activities require advanced reflexive knowledge both about the contents of work, such as new practices, clinical issues, technologies and machines, and about the organisational contexts of work.

Knowledge of the organisational context was particularly noted to by an English nurse, who even stated that knowledge about the health care system was a key component of a nurse's knowledge. Nurses' awareness of their various roles, status and also liabilities was indicated, more or less explicitly, in all cases. Irish nurses, for instance, discussed how awareness may, in general, be raised in the context of introducing new nursing roles. The new roles were seen as opportunities for raising the status of nursing, but also as harbouring risks. Indeed, some nurses were sceptical of being given new responsibilities without a discussion of legal changes and liabilities, which is another indication of high awareness about contexts. Our narrative data show that nurses were quite capable of doing reflexive self-analysis and putting their profession in the context of wider structural conditions.

Assuredly, these far-flung structural changes in health care have particular timings, directions and manifestations in different national contexts (Goodson and Norrie 2005; Beach 2005). Yet, we observed that regardless of particular changes in health care institutions, working conditions and management, they all seem to pose challenges to nurses' perceptions of their practice and knowledge in every country.

SYMBOLIC EXPRESSIONS OF SOCIAL ORGANISATION

In common parlance care means tending to the needs of another individual. Within the nursing profession, care is also seen as those distinctive features that distinguish nursing from the tasks of other health care staff. Our informants drew the strongest professional boundary around care in relation to the cure exercised by doctors. Nurses considered cure to be rooted in the bio-medical sciences and related knowledge. Another boundary was set against the non-professional caring and house-keeping tasks of the attendants (cf. Allen 1997; Dahle 2003; Davies 2003; Daykin and Clarke 2000). However, in reality nurses' work certainly includes occasional technical and bio-medical tasks, basic caring tasks, "paperwork" and caring of patients' "social context" (Carmel 2005). In general, care has both instrumental and expressive components (Woodward 1997), referring to manual and technical skills and knowledge, and social skills and psycho-socio-emotional knowledge. It is almost impossible to distinguish between technical and social skills in nursing practice. Therefore, the "unique" definition of nursing care as legitimate professional knowledge is embedded in this ambiguous relation concerning work also done by doctors and nursing assistants.

The multidisciplinary and combinatory as well as gendered character of nursing care and knowledge may be problematic in terms of perceiving it as proper professional knowledge. For instance, Davies (1995) has noted that there is a tension between the notion of the profession as rational, objective, autonomous and powerful, which is gendered masculine, and the central values of care, that are gendered feminine and psycho-emotional. Thus, there seems to be a strong tension between the traditional self-image and characterisation of nursing as psycho-socio-emotional knowledge and the traditional notions of professionalism. Many of our informants voiced this tension between objective-cum-scientific nursing and subjective-cum-emotional care. In addition, some participant nurses, for instance, one in the Spanish case, articulated the conflicting demands of being professionals and being women who do caring.

This ambiguity of representing nursing care was noticeable in our informants' almost simultaneous emphasis on nursing care as an innate, even un-learnable personal capacity, and their explicit calls for perceiving nursing as professional work and not only as women's work. It seems clear that within the conception of nursing care there inheres a tension between the personal (subjective and emotional) and professional (objective and intellectual). We can agree that to some extent nursing involves aspects of "emotional labour" (Hochschild 1983; Smith 1992), which tries to "influence patients' feelings." Yet, professional service as emotional labour can be contradictory in terms. Our data shows, however, that the above-mentioned tension between personal and professional also leads to attempts to balance these demands and limit the scope of the personal aspect of nursing, which we will discuss in a later section.

Nursing care, as a subject area of nurse training, was introduced into curricula from the establishment of nursing science as a critical and self-reflective discipline in the universities in the late 1970s and the early 1980s in Europe (Beach 2005). Nursing science consists of many disciplinary elements. Beckstead and Beckstead (2006) have conducted a citation analysis of scientific nursing journals revealing that the epistemic origins of nursing science cluster around three disciplinary groups, philosophy (nursing philosophy), social and psychological sciences and bio-medical sciences. Our participant nurses' perception of care and work tasks was, across contexts, with some variation, mainly two-fold, representing the division into instrumental and expressive components of care (Woodward 1997). Thus, care is internally organised by the same opposition that organises nurses' ideas about care (now humanistic and personal) in relation to cure (now bio-medical and technical) (cf. Bourdieu 1990, 177). The same division between technical and personal, or bio-medical and humanistic could be found in nurses' ideas about care reflecting the various epistemic sources of nursing science. Moreover, the classifications are not just purely cognitive but can also be used for evaluative purposes. For instance, in the Spanish context, a division was made between the "bad" nurses, who just apply technical nursing knowledge, and "good" ones, who integrate technical and medical knowledge and proper nursing care.

Nurses also attempted to overcome or bypass the previously cited oppositions. The ideas of multidisciplinary knowledge and holistic care have been introduced in nursing education and were also discussed by our informants. For instance, a Spanish nurse brought up an intermediary category, representing nurses in multidisciplinary and multi-professional contexts. The role of a mediator between patients and health care system can also be regarded as an attempt to overcome the opposition. Patient advocacy and a sort of a translator role between medical and lay knowledge were pointed to in many contexts as well. The comparisons of nurses' perceptions of caring in differing settings indicate that caring is a highly context-dependent conception (Bassett 2002; citing Greenhalgh et al. 1998). The fundamental oppositions between care and cure, and between instrumental (technical) and expressive (personal) care, structure the perceptions and judgments of our informants, but in various social conditions and relations these oppositions could achieve various articulations.

These mental oppositions, plucked from the data by the analyst, can be regarded as symbolic expression of the social organisation of health care (Durkheim 1965). They are parallel to the division of labour between nurses and doctors and the distribution of tasks within nursing. The fields of health care and nursing, like other social realities, have a twofold structure, consisting of the material reality of social organisation and the symbolic reality of discourse, meanings and representations (Bourdieu 1990, 135). Following Bourdieu (1981; 1990) we argue that mental classifications are embodied through professional socialisation into dispositions of agents and thereby organise actions, perceptions and judgements. Through practices dispositions produce structured outcomes in nurses' ideas about their work in which an analyst can observe homologous oppositions, such as "cure" versus "care", "technical" versus "personal", "biomedical" versus "humanistic", "task orientation" versus "whole patient", "biomedical machinery" and "human touch". These mental categories are not only related to the division of labour between doctors (who principally cure) and nurses (who principally care), but are also institutionalised into structures and practices of nursing science and education.

Why then do our informants' accounts contain illogicalities and inconsistencies? Structures of social field, such as the organisation of health care and nursing, are transformed into mental structures that are shared by the agents socialised into that social order. Thus, social structures and mental structures are parallel, but the former do not determine the latter completely because the social reality can be perceived from many different principles of classification. In addition, practical logic is always to an extent inconsistent and illogical. Practice aims at practical and not theoretical goals and is therefore only practically coherent; it is to some degree internally contradictory and fuzzy to an external observer. The principle of the minimum coherence required is "analogical practice founded on the *transfer of schemes*" (Bourdieu 2000, 54-7; 1990, 200-270). On the one hand, if social agents live in the same social conditions and through similar experiences, they "tend to perceive the social world according to the same principle of division which is objectified in a number of inevitable alternatives" (Bourdieu 2000, 83). On the other hand, because agents occupy different and opposing positions in the social space, they tend to "give opposing priority to each of the branches of the alternatives depending on the position they occupy in the structure" (ibid.). Nurses share the objective social reality with other health care professionals and staff, but have a distinctive social position and related point of view of the social organisation of the system.

Nurses tend to account for their own position as well as nursing care in different ways when representing it in relation to doctors compared to assistants or patients. The same nurse could practically define nursing care first as a personal and innate capability (in relation to doctors), and in the same interview few sentences later, as a skill based on nursing science (in relation to assistants and patients). For instance, in the Greek cases, it was perceivable that nurses emphasised their scientific training and higher educational qualifications in order to distinguish themselves, for instance, from the nursing assistants and more "traditional" nurses. On those occasions Greek nurses defined care as professional activity, based on a distinctive scientific knowledge and thus notably different from the on care activities of the nursing assistants. These findings are congruent with Dahle's (2003) observation that nurses have made "basic care" their exclusive preserve and, thus, try to distinguish their profession from the housewifely" activities of nursing assistants. However, Greek nurses also reported a widespread negative cultural attitude towards scientific knowledge and research among themselves. Moreover, in practice there was not always a clear differentiation between the tasks of the professional groups, which is attributable to the shortage of adequately qualified professional nurses. Sometimes nursing assistants are in charge in situations that would officially require a qualified nurse.

Educational variability adds to the diversity of roles and functions within nursing and force nurses to constantly negotiate the social order among their colleagues. The integration of nursing programmes into higher education institutions (see Goodson & Norries 2005; Beach 2005; Spitzer & Perrenoud 2006) has been a perceptible change across Europe. This has contributed to social relations at work, especially to that between "non-academic" senior nurses and "academic" junior nurses. These social oppositions have caused the tensions described by most informants. In many countries the introduction of academic education for nurses was greeted by the senior nurses and general public with great scepticism about the practical capabilities of the university-trained nurses and their willingness to get down to dirty work. On the other hand, some informants argued that younger nurses tend to treat patients holistically whereas older nurses are more oriented to tasks and techniques. Senior nurses often exercise peer control and supervision, but also offer valuable advice and informal training to junior nurses. The distinction between the theoretical (academic education) and practical (learning from experience) modes of knowledge underlies these relationships between the young and the old (see also Bassett 2002). Our data does not, however, show that there are real generational differences.

NURSING CARE, KNOWLEDGE AND ACCOUNTABILITY

One important aspect of the restructuring of welfare state services has been that welfare professionals, such as nurses and doctors, are increasingly being held accountable for their work. Professionals need to meet efficiency targets and apply standardised models at work, devise strategies, document their activities and be open to periodical evaluations. Today, the idea of personal responsibility and accountability is even introduced to nurses in education programmes (see Apesoa-Varano 2007).

Evidence-based[i] nursing and current care guidelines are types of standardised models for work, which were frequently brought up by the nurses in our interviews. In this context nursing care was not discussed in terms of the "personal touch" anymore, but as an objective and legitimate procedure. Nurses were unanimous

[i] For more about social science perspectives on evidence-based medicine, see special issue in Social Science & Medicine 2006, 62 (10). 'Evidence' and evidence-based medicine can be problematised and challenged from the post-positivist, feminist and phenomenological philosophies of science (see Goldenberg 2006).

in the fact that their work procedures should be based on state-of-the-art medicine and nursing. Many informants regarded evidence-based practice as a crucial feature of their self-reflexive work and perceive blind routine practice as contrary to it. However, evidence-based practice may not be totally unproblematic in all circumstances as it seems to be a peculiar combination of autonomous professional activity and accountability based on established guidelines. Evidence-based practice can be perceived both in terms of gaining autonomy and losing it at the same time. It defines, on the one hand, a special sphere of activity for nurses, but, on the other hand, those activities are defined by externally imposed standards. Still, nurses mainly embrace the guidelines because they respond to their quest for clarity in liability.

Walby et al. (1994) suggest that the nurses' approach to evidence-based practice and clinical decision-making is different from doctors' individual, informed decision-making. Nurses often perceive evidence-based practice precisely in terms of its effect on ensuring safety and accountability. Evidence-based practice is viewed as a means of dealing collectively with risks. For instance, the Swedish nurses talk about losing control when there are no standardised procedures or tools available. The Finnish nurses also emphasised "doing everything right, according to current knowledge". Thus, "using one's knowledge right" and "knowing one's limits" were significant features of work. Responsibility and accuracy were strongly emphasised across the cases.

It seems that even though nurses talk about care as the "human touch", their professional judgement is rooted in standardised modes of operation and collective accountability rather than on the art of individual professional judgement and accountability (MacDonald 1995, 164-5). The latter mode of professional judgment has been more prevalent among doctors. This is in all likelihood linked to the organisation of work, the primordial element of which is an individual doctor's appointment, and the art of diagnosis. However, nowadays doctors' work is also guided more and more by external models of current care and best practice. Nevertheless, recent research shows that even doctors in managerial positions seem to rely more on individual professional experience than guidelines (Viitanen et al. 2006). Professional practice is usually regarded in literature as excluding personal emotions. If caring is strongly regarded as personal and emotional work, then this will cause ambiguity in the professional and social status of nurses. (MacDonald 1995, 137). When nurses talked about evidence-based care, however, they no longer attached emotions to their accounts. They were more concerned about the application of valid procedures and the potential liabilities involved.

Because nurses refer to their practice more as a functional whole rather than as an individual enterprise related to individual achievements and talent, then perhaps we should organise nurses' professional accountability in collective terms as well. The current conception of professional work, the prototype of being a lawyer or doctor, may not fit well with nurses' professional culture and its dominating institutions. Indeed, the nurses themselves express the problem of reconciling their collective ambitions rooted in care and in their striving to be recognised as respected professionals (Degeling et al. 2000). In fact, present-day regulations seem to imply some sort of shared accountability and would therefore fit quite well with nurses' professional self-understanding and the organisation of their practice in groups. Indeed, our case studies reported few instances where physicians seemed to actually have more difficulties in adapting to the new regulations, guidelines and modes of operation, such as multi-professional teams. Though these references were few, they illustrated, on the one hand, how nurses negotiate the appropriate nursing care in terms of common sets of rules and regulations, and blame doctors for not being adaptive and responsive to them. On the other hand, these instances showed actual difficulties that some doctors may have in adapting to the new modes of operation redefining their professional autonomy and professionalism as based on independent clinical decision-making and individual accountability (Viitanen et al. 2006; Walby et al. 1994).

DEFINING THE LIMITS AND CONTENT OF NURSING CARE

Our interview data show two main fronts in which nurses try to limit their scope of practice and responsibility. First, they try to maintain a boundary between personal and professional aspects of work, which is an ambiguous goal since at the same time they want to differentiate their work from doctors' work by emphasising its emotional and subjective aspects. Second, nurses need to negotiate daily with other occupational groups, such as doctors and nursing assistants, about the proper division of tasks and duties. Other studies have also reported that the division of work between nurses and doctors is not fixed but flexibly distributed (see Allen 1997; Goodwin et al. 2005).

Health care policy is increasingly concerned with efficiency and accountability. An ever greater amount of clinical guidelines have been introduced. Medical science and technology have opened new opportunities in therapy and treatment not witnessed before. Yet the core of nurses' occupational identity seems to be still defined according to patient care (Kirpal 2003). Indeed, this area of focus may have even strengthened, having a central position in nursing education and ideology.[ii] Pelttari (1997) explained how in Finland the "human-to-human" requirements have been the focus since the inception of nurse's training in polytechnics in the early 1990s. Nursing science has, since its establishment, also been producing substantial research on human relations. These dominant voices were echoed by the Finnish informants, who highlight nurses having "sensitive radar", or "a certain touch" with people. Nevertheless, the very same nurses also emphasised the need to keep a distance from patients and maintain the nurse's professional stance towards patients as important aspects of professional skills. It seems that these Finnish nurses try to find

[ii] Quotation from the Finnish Nurses Association's presentation: "Nurses have their patient's needs foremost at heart." (p. 2) http://www.sairaanhoitajaliitto.fi/mp/db/file_library/x/IMG/49439/file/SSL_yleisesite_engl_4.pdf [Accessed September 22, 2008]

a balance between the meeting patients' needs, as they perceive it, and maintaining a professional distance, role and status. In the Finnish context, nurses' professionalism was strongly connected to an awareness of the limits of nursing practice, while in other contexts, e.g. in Greece, the line between a personal and professional, though scientific base of nursing was emphasised in other occasions, was perhaps not as clear as in Finland. In Spain the line between personal and professional was even more problematic for the nurses, as they saw a tension between "being a nurse" and "working as a nurse". This observation approaches Dyson's (1996) on how nurses perceived caring as a combination of what the nurses do and what the nurses are like as persons. The nurse's work style was found to be a key component in regard to the former, and sensitivity, giving of one's self, and the nurse's general approach portrayed the latter.

While maintaining more or less close personal relations with the patients can be stressful, it also has many obviously advantages. Close relations to patients and the informal extra-medical knowledge that is obtained through communication with them can be used for constructing and securing a distinctive professional position within the field of health care. For instance, nurses in the Finnish context described clients as important sources of knowledge, because they are "the experts of their own health". This statement implies the undermining of doctors' authority that is based on their expertise in medical science and diagnostics. Furthermore, it is linked to nurses' efforts to secure a role as a patient advocate and/or a mediator between patients and the health care system. The short quotation, however, also echoes the present-day discourse of consumerism and patients' rights. Although English nurses were often irritated by too demanding and rights-conscious patients, they were also very concerned about losing the informal knowledge derived directly from communication with patients in informal situations due to outsourcing of various services, such as catering.

We have to bear in mind that although nurses highlight care, listening, comforting and expressing sensitivity, it is not self-evident that the patients share this enthusiasm. Indeed, Bassett (2002) has interestingly pointed out that the patients actually prefer competent and technical nursing skills and abilities to expressive humanistic behaviour. Yet, our informants often seem to assume that patients are concerned more with the expressive rather than instrumental aspects of care.

The demarcation of nursing from other health care occupations was well illustrated by a Portuguese nurse who said that she lost the essential part of being a nurse, that is "bedside nursing", a "part of [her] professional fulfilment", when she moved into management. Another Portuguese nurse described her work in outpatient care as such that could be done by a technician: "I am not a technician, a lab technician, I am a nurse." She saw outpatient care as limited in scope, merely work suitable for medical practice assistants. She preferred working in a health centre because she felt more "nurse-like" there. We can observe two things here. First, the nurse's perception of preferred nursing and nurse-like activity is continuous activity, involving a close, trusting relationship with patients, and attending to their needs in an organisation with other health care staff. Second, a distinction is made between two kinds of caring activities, and the technician's role is attributed to nursing assistants. As mentioned above, Dahle (2003) has similarly observed similarly how nurses make themselves distinct from assistants, even though in practice both occupations are involved in overlapping caring tasks. Furthermore, in her study (ibid.), the nursing assistants emphasised the practical nature of the work of both nurses' and themselves. They stressed similarities between the two groups while the nurses focused upon the differences.

Efforts to limit the content and scope of nursing practice in relation to other occupational groups were evident in the Irish context, too. An interesting instance was reported where a nurse refused to carry out a certain procedure despite the entreaty of a junior doctor. The doctor's request and the nurse's refusal could also be seen in terms of a differential understanding of accountability by these two professional groups as described above (see also Walby et al. 1994). This individual event indicated how nurses tend to rely on collective accountability and concern for liability whereas doctors perceive their professional judgement as an individual decision for which they are individually accountable (see also Degeling et al. 2000). Consequently, nurses' inflexibility can be misunderstood by the doctors, much as the doctors' activities can be misunderstood by the nurses. This difference could be an indication of a difference in professional ethos, but it could also be related to social status and/or the gendered history of these professions. These differences might be changing as medical work is more often organised around teams and standardised models of evidence-based medicine and current care guidelines diffuse across the field.

As we have shown, the division between care and cure and the various definitions of care are loaded with ambiguities. Our informants, however, also made efforts to go beyond these ambiguities or tried to combine these oppositions. That is, nurses may vacillate between "technical" and "personal" aspects of their knowledge and work, but they may also try to establish an overarching category of "holistic care", or "interdisciplinary knowledge" that combines the medical and humanistic domains of knowledge. This effort is also echoed in nurses' ideas about their efforts to obtain an intermediary role between the health care system and patients. For instance, in the Spanish case a nurse was seen as "an interconnecting node between whole networks of health professionals", translating the expert medical discourse to a non-expert patient with a limited knowledge of medicine.

The role of an advocate for patients and a mediator between lay and medical knowledge was highlighted by most of our informants. This easiness to adopt the role of mediator could be understood by the fact that nurse's knowledge, their point of view and language, does not presuppose such a clear-cut break with common sense. In contrast, the doctor's diagnostic point of view on illness presupposes a total break with common sense, and thus means that the patient does not only confront a different language, but also a totally different way of constructing the given illness (Bourdieu 2000, 57-8).

Although nurses may try to break down the division between "technical" and "human", and have actually managed go beyond it to a degree by such formulations as holistic care, they are still quite eager to attach distinctive attributes to these fundamental categories. For instance, Spanish nurses were quite extreme in rendering knowledge of care as a personal quality or pre-disposition that cannot be learned. In contrast, technical and medical knowledge is seen as learnable by everyone. Spanish nurses describe care as "heart", "personal attitude", the "human touch in the face of bio-medical machinery", highlighting the distinction between emotional-cum-personal care and objectifying impersonal treatment.

NURSING CARE AND RESTRUCTURING

Our informants talked very much about the social and material conditions of work, such as work overload, haste, limited time and human resources, when they addressed their practice. They paid much attention to the managerial, administrative and structural changes of health care, which contribute to the possibilities of realising the ideas and knowledge they have learned in education and at work, and of generating new ideas and knowledge.

Tight budgets and administrative steering in health care settings have two important consequences on nursing care. First, the lack of resources and managerial support makes both applying and learning nursing care knowledge problematic. Second, the context of high flexibility and heavy staff rotation makes continuing knowledge acquisition crucial. These conditions often make learning autodidactic and on-the-job. Nurses in most study contexts emphasised "a continuous need to stay informed, and to personally investigate and keep up to date" with current practices. This was an important concern of their professional practice, regardless of the real opportunities or incentives available. The idea of the holistic approach, which is very demanding, might actually lead to frustration at work because the ideal is not easily realised in the given structural and material conditions. There might not be time and human resources to provide personal care or apply up-to-date clinical guidelines. Consequently, nurses may find it hard to clarify the scope and limits of their professional activity to themselves and others in conditions of shortages or conflicting demands (cf. Attree 2005; McGillis Hall & Kiesners 2005).

The nurses' emphasis on constant learning and knowledge acquisition can be seen as more than a mere expression of actual needs in everyday work. Nurses often connect "keeping up to date with things" to the quality patient care which is at the core of their professional self-understanding and identity. Furthermore, and most interestingly, what they mean by "keeping up to date" refers usually to the models of current practices and guidelines. Furthermore, while nurses talk about a personal responsibility to keep up to date, their responses also imply some sort of collective learning because guidelines are understood by nurses as a means to be accountable as a group (Walby et al. 1994). Nurses keep up to date with a common set of practices, regulations, instructions and modes of operation in order to provide proper patient care. "Things" with which they keep up to date are not individual ways of thinking, problem-solving or decision-making, but rather sets of rules and codes of conduct. Yet, they are also able to see that outdated and rigid guidelines may become obstacles to professional development and innovation.

CONCLUSION

Caring is often defined as providing physical, spiritual, emotional and social comfort to patients. It is regarded by many as the core of nurses' professional identification (Bassett 2002; Kirpal 2003) and the main motivation to enter and remain in the profession. We have tried to show on the basis of interviews in seven European countries that nursing care is a very ambiguous idea and practice, which is practised and discussed in a variety of ways depending on the social relations and conditions in which it is embedded. The system of scientific and explicit knowledge of nursing care, produced in nursing science and passed on in nursing education and professional journals, is used as the basis for the claims for particular expertise. Scientifically established nursing care distinguishes nurses from other health care occupations, particularly from nursing assistants and lay people. Yet, in relation to medical doctors nurses tend to emphasise the humanistic aspects of their work.

We have not tried to find more logic and consistency in our informants' ideas than there actually is. The more explicit and systematic model – the fundamental division between care and cure, the parallel sub-categories of technical and personal, and bio-medical and humanistic, and their relation to the division of labour in health care – presented here is an analytic device provided by us in order to understand the diverse accounts of our informants.

Health care is currently becoming more and more dominated by science, technology and economy. Therefore public expectations involve much more than the mere "human touch". This puts nurses in a complex situation seeking the right balance between the bio-medical and humanistic aspects of their work. While health care is becoming more dependent on bio-medicine and medical technology and regulated by stricter managerial control, nurses try to overcome the distinction between the technical and humanistic by means of such notions as holistic and interdisciplinary care.

Undoubtedly, people have always been the focus of nurses' work. However, this orientation is by no means unproblematic in the current concerns of cost, efficiency and technology. The experience of haste and shortage of staff makes it difficult to concentrate on caring for the patients, that is, spending time with them and giving them psychological and social support. Nurses often argue that they have only time to do "bio-medical tricks". Furthermore, it is not only the psycho-social side of nursing that is jeopardised by the existing conditions. Nurses also say that it is sometimes even difficult to achieve the standards of current care models required by management.

The domain of nurses' professional knowledge and practice is not exhausted in the classifications of cure and care, technical and personal, or bio-medical and humanistic. We want to briefly mention another increasingly important domain, which is becoming more and more central in health care organisations, namely that of administration, management and organisation of work. This domain of knowledge has become particularly important because various ideas of decentralisation, self-organisation and self-management have been put forward by new health care policies that try to render the system more efficient. Nowadays, nurses are urged to be self-regulative agents who plan, innovate, execute, monitor and evaluate their own work. In the present conditions of cost-efficiency and scarcity, however, there are potential problems in the self-management and self-organisation of health care units. Nurses often have to improvise and devise new solutions to practical problems in conditions like a shortage of qualified staff, strict organisational orders, distorted communication channels and slow decision-making procedures.

We have shown in this article that nursing work is not just emotional labour or patient-centred care, but contains many technical, bio-medical and administrative tasks as well. Furthermore, nursing encompasses manifold roles and functions in various settings. We think it is time to retreat from defining nursing purely around patient care, distinct from the activities of other health care professionals. Instead we should examine more carefully what nurses and other health care personnel actually do at work and how material and symbolic resources and conditions provide opportunities and set constraints on their ambitions.

REFERENCES

Allen, D. (1997). The Nursing-Medical Boundary: A Negotiated Order? *Sociology of Health and Illness*, 19(4), 498-520.

Apesoa-Varano E. C. (2007). Educated Caring: The Emergence of Professional Identity among Nurses. *Qualitative Sociology*, 30(3), 249-274.

Arts, W. & Gelissen, J. (2002). Three Worlds of Welfare Capitalism or More? A State-of-the Art Report. *Journal of European Social Policy*, 12(2), 137-158.

Attree, M. (2005). Nursing Agency and Governance: Registered Nurses' Perceptions. *Journal of Nursing Management*, 13(5), 387-396.

Bassett, Chris. 2002. Nurses' Perception of Care and Caring. *International Journal of Nursing Practice*, 8(1), 8-15.

Beach B., Ed. (2005) *Work-package 2: Welfare State Restructuring in Education and Health Care: Implications for the Teaching and Nursing Professions and their Professional Knowledge*. Deliverable 2 in the EU Sixth Framework Programme Project Professional Knowledge in Education and Health: Restructuring Work and Life between the State and the Citizens in Europe. http://www.profknow.net/files/results/WP2.pdf. [Accessed June 2, 2008]

Beckstead, J. M. & Beckstead, L. G. (2006). A Multidimensional Analysis of the Epistemic Origins of Nursing Theories, Models, and Frameworks. *International Journal of Nursing Studies*, 43(1), 113-122.

Bourdieu, P. (2000). *Pascalian Meditations*. Cambridge: Polity Press.

Bourdieu, P. (1990). *The Logic of Practice*. Stanford: Stanford University Press.

Bourdieu, P. (1981). Men and Machines. In K. D. Knorr-Cetina and A. V. Cicourel (Eds.) *Advances in Social Theory and Methodology. Toward an Integration of Micro- and Macro-Sociology*. Boston: Routledge & Kegan Paul, 304-317.

Bryant-Lukosius, D., Dicenso, D. A., Browne, G. & Pinelli, J. (2004). Advanced Practice Nursing Roles: Development, Implementation and Evaluation. *Journal of Advanced Nursing*, 48(5), 519-529.

Carmel, S. (2005). Health Care Practices, Professions and Perspectives: A Case Study in Intensive Care. *Social Science & Medicine*, 62(8), 2079-2090.

Dahle, R. (2003). Shifting Boundaries of Negotiations on Knowledge: Interprofessional Conflicts between Nurses and Nursing Assistants in Norway. *International Journal of Sociology and Social Policy*, 23(4/5), 129-158.

Davies, C. (1995). Competence versus Care? Gender and Caring Work Revisited. *Acta Sociologica*, 38(1), 17-31.

Davies, K. (2003). The Body and Doing Gender: The Relations between Doctors and Nurses in Hospital Work. *Sociology of Health & Illness*, 25(7), 720–742.

Daykin, N. & Clarke, B. (2000). 'They'll Still Get the Bodily Care'. Discourses of Care and Relationships between Nurses and Health Care Assistants in the NHS. *Sociology of Health & Illness*, 22(3), 349–363.

Degeling, P., Hill, M., Kennedy, J., Coyle, B. & Maxwell, S. (2000). A Cross-National Study of Differences in the Identities of Nursing in England and Australia and How This Has Affected Nurses' Capacity to Respond to Hospital Reform. *Nursing Inquiry*, 7(2), 120-135.

Dupont, M. & Sugrue, C. (2007). Irish Nurses' Work and Life under Restructuring: Professional Experiences, Knowledge and Expertise in Changing Contexts. In T. Kosonen & J. Houtsonen (Eds.) *European Nurses' Life and Work under Restructuring: Professional Experiences, Knowledge and Expertise in Changing Context*. Deliverable 5 in the EU Sixth Framework Programme Project Professional Knowledge in Education and Health: Restructuring Work and Life between the State and the Citizens in Europe, 89-146. http://www.profknow.net/files/results/D05_European_Nurses_Life_and_Work_under_Restructuring.pdf. [Accessed June 3, 2008]

Durkheim, E. (1965). *The Elementary Forms of the Religious Life*. New York: Free Press.

Dyson, J. (1996). Nurses' Conceptualisations of Caring Attitudes and Behaviours. *Journal of Advanced Nursing*, 23(6), 1263–1269.

Goldenberg, M. J. (2006). On Evidence and Evidence-Based Medicine: Lessons from the Philosophy of Science. *Social Science & Medicine*, 62(11), 2621-2632.

Goodson, I. & Norrie, C. Eds. (2005). *A Literature Review of Welfare State Restructuring in Education and Health Care in European Contexts: Implications for the Teaching and Nursing Professions and Their Professional Knowledge*. Deliverable 1 in the EU Sixth Framework Programme Project Professional Knowledge in Education and Health: Restructuring Work and Life between the State and the Citizens in Europe. http://www.profknow.net/files/results/Literature_Review_WP1_EU.pdf. [Accessed June 16, 2008]

Goodwin, D., Pope, C., Mort, M. & Smith, A. (2005). Access, Boundaries and Their Effects: Legitimate Participation in Anaesthesia. *Sociology of Health & Illness*, 27(6), 855-871.

Greenhalgh, J., Vanhanen, L. & Kyngäs, H. (1998). Nurse Caring Behaviours. *Journal of Advanced Nursing*, 27(5), 927–932.

Hochschild, Arlie. 1983. *The Managed Heart: The Commercialization of Human Feeling*. Berkeley: University of California Press.

Kirpal, S. (2003). *Nurses in Europe. Work Identities of Nurses across 4 European Countries*. University of Bremen: Institute of Technology and Education. ITB – Forschungsberichte 07/2003. http://www.itb.uni-bremen.de/downloads/Publikationen/Forschungsberichte/FB_07_03.pdf. [Accessed June 3, 2008]

Kosonen, T. & Houtsonen, J. Eds. (2007a). *European Nurses' Life and Work under Restructuring: Professional Experiences, Knowledge and Expertise in Changing Context*. Deliverable 5 in the EU Sixth Framework Programme Project Professional Knowledge in Education and Health: Restructuring Work and Life between the State and the Citizens in Europe. http://www.profknow.net/files/results/D05_European_Nurses_Life_and_Work_under_Restructuring.pdf. [Accessed June 3, 2008]

Kosonen, T. & Houtsonen, J. (2007b). Finnish Nurses. In T. Kosonen & J. Houtsonen (Eds.) *European Nurses' Life and Work under Restructuring: Professional Experiences, Knowledge and Expertise in Changing Context*. Deliverable 5 in the EU Sixth Framework Programme Project Professional Knowledge in Education and Health: Restructuring Work and Life between the State and the Citizens in Europe, 259-279. http://www.profknow.net/files/results/D05_European_Nurses_Life_and_Work_under_Restructuring.pdf. [Accessed June 3, 2008].

Macdonald, K. M. 1995. *The Sociology of Professions*. London: Sage.

McGillis Hall, L. & Kiesners, D. (2005). A Narrative Approach to Understanding the Nursing Work Environment in Canada. *Social Science & Medicine*, 61(12), 2482-2491.

Müller, J., Larrain V., Creus, A., Marrero, I., Muntadas, M., Hernándes, F. & Sancho Gil, J. M. (2007). Case Study Report Life Histories – Nurses Spain. In T. Kosonen & J. Houtsonen (Eds.) *European Nurses' Life and Work under Restructuring: Professional Experiences, Knowledge and Expertise in Changing Context*. Deliverable 5 in the EU Sixth Framework Programme Project Professional Knowledge in Education and Health: Restructuring Work and Life between the State and the Citizens in Europe, 199-226. http://www.profknow.net/files/results/D05_European_Nurses_Life_and_Work_under_Restructuring.pdf. [Accessed June 3, 2008]

Nancarrow, S. S. & Borthwick, A. M. (2005). Dynamic Professional Boundaries in the Healthcare Workforce. *Sociology of Health & Illness*, 27(7), 897-919.

Norrie, C. & Goodson, I. (2007). English Nurses' Work and Life under Restructuring: Professional Experiences, Knowledge and Expertise in Changing Contexts. In T. Kosonen & J. Houtsonen (Eds.) *European Nurses' Life and Work under Restructuring: Professional Experiences, Knowledge and Expertise in Changing Context*. Deliverable 5 in the EU Sixth Framework Programme Project Professional Knowledge in Education and Health: Restructuring Work and Life between the State and the Citizens in Europe, 61-88. http://www.profknow.net/files/results/D05_European_Nurses_Life_and_Work_under_Restructuring.pdf. [Accessed June 3, 2008]

Pelttari, P. (1997). *Sairaanhoitajan työn nykyiset ja tulevaisuuden kvalifikaatiovaatimukset*. Tutkimuksia 80. Helsinki. Stakes.

Pereira, H. (2007). Portuguese Nurses' Work and Life under Restructuring: Professional Experiences, Knowledge and Expertise in Changing Contexts. In T. Kosonen & J. Houtsonen (Eds.) *European Nurses' Life and Work under Restructuring: Professional Experiences, Knowledge and Expertise in Changing Context*. Deliverable 5 in the EU Sixth Framework Programme Project Professional Knowledge in Education and Health: Restructuring Work and Life between the State and the Citizens in Europe, 169-198. http://www.profknow.net/files/results/D05_European_Nurses_Life_and_Work_under_Restructuring.pdf. [Accessed June 3, 2008]

Rantalaiho, L. (2004). Loppusanat. In L. Henriksson & S. Wrede (Eds.) *Hyvinvointityön ammatit*. Helsinki. Gaudeamus.

Safilou-Rothschild, C. (2007). Greek Nurses' Work and Life under Restructuring: Professional Experiences, Knowledge and Expertise in Changing Contexts. In T. Kosonen & J. Houtsonen (Eds.) *European Nurses' Life and Work under Restructuring: Professional Experiences, Knowledge and Expertise in Changing Context*. Deliverable 5 in the EU Sixth Framework Programme Project Professional Knowledge in Education and Health: Restructuring Work and Life between the State and the Citizens in Europe, 147-168. http://www.profknow.net/files/results/D05_European_Nurses_Life_and_Work_under_Restructuring.pdf. [Accessed June 3, 2008]

Smith, P. 1992. *Emotional Labour of Nursing*. Hampshire: Palgrave Macmillan.

Spitzer, A., & Perrenoud, B. (2006). Reforms in Nursing Education across Western Europe: Implementation Processes and Current Status. *Journal of Professional Nursing*, 22(3), 162-171.

Viitanen, E., Lehto J., Tampsi-Jarvala T., Mattila, K., Virjo, I., Isokoski, M., Hyyppölä, H., Kumpusalo, E., Halila, H., Kujala, S. & Vänskä, J. (2006) Doctor-managers as Decision Makers in Hospitals and Health Centres. *Journal of Health Organization and Management*, 20(2), 85-94.

Walby, S., Greenwell, J., MacKay, L. & Soothill, K. (1994). *Medicine and Nursing: Professions in a Changing Health Service*. London: Sage.

Woodward, V. M. (1997). Professional Caring: A Contradiction in Terms? *Journal of Advanced Nursing*, 26(5), 999-1004.

Wärvik, G.-B. (2007). Nurses' Life Histories: The Swedish Case. In T. Kosonen & J. Houtsonen (Eds.) *European Nurses' Life and Work under Restructuring: Professional Experiences, Knowledge and Expertise in Changing Context*. Deliverable 5 in the EU Sixth Framework Programme Project Professional Knowledge in Education and Health: Restructuring Work and Life between the State and the Citizens in Europe, 227-258. http://www.profknow.net/files/results/D05_European_Nurses_Life_and_Work_under_Restructuring.pdf. [Accessed June 3, 2008]

ISAAC MARRERO & JÖRG MÜLLER

NEW MANAGEMENT, CONTROL AND AUTONOMY

INTRODUCTION

New Public Management has been one of the critical strategies of restructuring welfare institutions such as education and health care. It has meant the introduction of various measures of cost-control and accountability. It has also changed, when considered together with the process of professionalization, the boundaries between professions and the distribution of authority and responsibility. In this chapter we will look at the ways these transformations have affected nurses, particularly at the level of everyday work and in relation to their autonomy and control. In this sense, we will explore an apparent paradox between increasing autonomy and increasing control. Our argument is that this dual process is not necessarily a paradox: nurses can be at once more autonomous and more controlled – precisely because changes in management have redefined these terms.

New Public Management (NPM) can be characterized in general terms as the introduction of market logic into the non-market public sector (Pollitt & Bouckaert 2005). Subdued to the regulating force of the market, so-called inefficient public services are forced to improve their internal workings in order to gain consumers' choice in a quest for the best service as well as to increase efficiency and streamline public administration. A whole battery of NPM instruments are at disposal to this effect, starting from open competition to private-sector management styles to standards for measuring performance and payment-by-result schemes (Harlow 2002). In health care, NPM has meant a focus on the consumer, an increase in efficiency concerns and a reliance on the notion of managerialism, all aimed at creating cost effective service provision and quality conscious health care workers (Bolton 2004). NPM is also linked to decentralization of management to local levels, that is, local institutions and individuals (Pollitt et al. 1998). These are, however, general traits that fail to grasp the great deal of variations present in each context. One of the aims of this chapter is, in fact, to show the particularities of the countries studied. In order to engage with those differences we have focused in the most salient features of NPM in each case. Instead of attempting to generalize, this chapter looks at the impact of accountability as seen most extremely (England and Ireland), the role technology plays in restructuring (Sweden), the redistribution of responsibility (Finland) and various forms of resistance to reform (Spain, Greece, Portugal).

With respect to 'autonomy', we have approached it at two levels: everyday work and administration. The former refers to nurses' control over tasks and duties at work; the latter refers to nurses' control over organization and management. Since

J. Houtsonen, G.-B. Wärvik (Eds.), European Nurses' Life and Work Under Restructuring pp. 77-94.

a significant dimension of autonomy is the possibility to participate in decision-making, we have looked at both clinical and administrative decision-making. The former implies some kind of professional judgements; the latter requires certain forms of collective organization. For both levels, autonomy can be attained formally (through legislation, agreements, etc.) and/or informally, gained and claimed through daily practices without official coverage. The general trend we have identified is that NPM, together with the redistribution of tasks and authority within the nursing profession and between nurses and doctors, have increased nurses' autonomy of *doing* but not their autonomy of *governing*. Nurses have increased their control over nursing and caring tasks and duties at work, but have not gained significant control over administration and management. There are, however, relevant particularities and exemptions across the national cases.

As for 'control', our use of the term in this chapter refers to a wide array of devices of subjection: human, technological, externally enforced, self-imposed, and collectively agreed. We will look at the impact of accountability, cost-control, guidelines for procedures, documentation protocols, peer evaluation, patients' complaints, software, etc. in nurses' professional practice. In accordance to NPM strategies, direct means of control and/or work supervision have in general been replaced by more indirect and less hierarchical forms. Control takes the form of target setting; peer-evaluation and self-management are equally fostered as more desirable architectures of authority; an efficient use of resources (material, time, financial, etc.) is monitored and encouraged by detailed accountability schemes. Here again, there is a general trend towards the introduction of instruments subduing health care to the logic of the market (therefore subjecting the provision of health care to economic criteria and targets), but several important differences were observed in the countries studied. Not only between the devices of control that were introduced, but among the impact they had had in actual everyday practices. The gap between the ideas (and practices) of change and the change in ideas (and practices) is one not to be overlooked.

THE PRESSURE OF ACCOUNTABILITY

A central technology for implementing accountability measures is documentation. There is a widespread agreement on the fact that paperwork and the need for documentation has increased over the past years. This not only is evident throughout the case studies but also in the survey: 75% of Finnish nurses, 91% of Irish nurses and 78 % of Swedish nurses agreed strongly on the fact that the demand of written documentation had increased (Sohlberg et al. 2007, 152). In a move to increase quality and efficiency of public care, an avalanche of guidelines and targets frame nursing work. This is especially apparent in England, the spearhead of neo-liberal restructuring in the EU, where nurses have to respond to National Frameworks, National Institute for Clinical Excellence (NICE) guidelines and ward inspections by the Health Commission. In a similar fashion, the Irish nurses mentioned the recent introduction of the Nursing and Midwifery Practice Framework (ABA,

2000) as having had a huge impact. The increased need for documentation derives from increased accountability towards patients/clients, the public, supervising or regulatory bodies, and their employers. Two accountability domains appeared as especially relevant in their implications for nurses' work conditions in the Irish[1] and English[2] case studies (Norrie & Goodson 2007; Dupont & Sugrue 2007).

Firstly, nurses were held accountable both legally and professionally for their care work. Different guidelines and quality frameworks in place defined the scope of nurses' responsibilities and obligations. The *Essence of Care* benchmarks introduced in 2001 by the National Institute for Clinical Excellence in England cover eight areas: continence, bladder and bowel care, personal hygiene, food and nutrition, pressure ulcers, privacy and dignity, record keeping, safety of patients with mental health needs, and principles of self care. In order to demonstrate that these standards had been met, nurses had to provide written evidence. This paperwork proved to be crucial since it provided evidence in relation to career promotion schemes, decisions in insurance matters or legal responsibilities among others. In Ireland nurses had to be prepared to make explicit the rationale for decisions they made and to justify such decisions in the context of legislation, professional standards and guidelines, evidence based practice, and professional and ethical rules of conduct. Irish and English nurses alike mentioned in this context the fear of litigation. In Ireland half of the nurses thought that there was a high risk of being sued (Sohlberg et al. 2007, 164). Since patients were becoming increasingly ready to resort to litigation nurses were highly aware of the need to document compliance with professional guidelines and legal constraints. One Irish nurse graphically illustrated how the need for documentation had changed. She recalled how early on her nursing career if someone fell out of the bed they were dusted off helped back in and asked if they wanted a cup of tea. Nowadays there was a whole procedure to be followed:

> Documentation must be filled out, insurance people informed, risk management informed, families informed. It's all what should be happening but it's a time-consuming, lengthy process. (Irish nurse 1)

[1] The Irish case study was based in a located within one of the networks of the Health Services Executive. It has over 600 beds and provides 24 hour service for an area of approximately 250.000 inhabitants. It is one of the busiest in the country, with an average bed occupancy rate of 100%. The hospital has also a strong academic dimension: it is the principal undergraduate and post-graduate medical training and research centre attached to a college of medicine and houses its own undergraduate and post graduate nurse training school. The hospital is managed by a Board of Management nominated by the Department of Health & Children, which also provides the funding. Its main priority is the treatment of public patients, but there are a number of beds reserved for private and semi-private patients.

[2] The study was based in a hospital in the South of England, part of a NHS Trust that provides general and specialist to a population of 500.000 and has around 5.000 members of staff. The hospital recently became a teaching hospital with a new medical school being attached to the Trust. The Trust had been poorly rated by the Health Care Commission and was in debt of over £10 million. This had led to staff redundancies and the introduction of a severe performativity agenda.

Similarly, an English nurse left little doubt about the importance of documentation:

> I feel it is all very important. Documentation has to be water-tight because I have done a law module for a medical, I mean I think that it has to be because, um, you have to be squeaky clean both on paper and on verbal and non-verbal; it's as simple as that. (English nurse 1)

Secondly, nurses were also financially accountable for the resources they used. They had to justify 'every ha'penny' of the temporal or material resources they used – as one of the Irish nurses put it. A financial controller monitored the work of Irish nurses and she had to provide temporary budgets every week. Since hospitals were also eager to reduce costs, nurses were expected to keep costs at a minimum. This in turn increased paperwork. In the English hospital every procedure or intervention had to be documented and fed into a central system to work out its costs. With the splitting of accounting systems into the public NHS and private insurances this became an especially tedious administrative task.

At this point the Swedish case study becomes illustrative. It allows us to describe in greater detail the implications of informatization of nurses' work. Technology has been an important tool in the introduction of new management strategies. Information and communication technologies (ICT), to various extents, have helped shaping the process of restructuration by providing the technical means necessary for certain policies to be implemented. ICT can neither be globally rejected nor hailed as improving or deteriorating nurses' work. Rather, there are several factors that influence how technology impacts on professional autonomy and control of nurses.

THE USES OF TECHNOLOGY

One of the key contributions of ICT to management has been the possibility of building centralized and standardized information systems. These systems gather and sort massive amounts of information in an accessible way. They have been instrumental in a more fluent administration of patient files, for example. They have also opened new channels of communication and sharing of information between professionals. They, too, have provided a platform for detailed measuring of performance, efficiency, costs, etc. ICT, then, have fostered new dynamics at various levels – and we will try to preserve this complexity when commenting on them.

The power of technological infrastructure as an actor channelling the daily routine of nurses was apparent in our study of a primary health care centre in Göteborg, Sweden[3] (Wärvik 2007). The development of a comprehensive computerized system was in this case as much a tool for facilitating general procedures and communication

[3] The Centre is located in an urban, multicultural, relatively impoverished area. It employs around 60 professionals, ten of which are nurses. It is run by the regional council and it belongs to the public health care system, even if, as we will see, it is funded by a 'purchasing scheme' that reimburses costs according to achievements. The supervisor and the assistant supervisor of the Centre are both nurses, as it is the area manager.

among professionals as a tool for the linking of health care and economic goals. For example, one of the main tasks of nurses in the Centre was distributing the patients. Before they could be treated, nurses had to assess the situation of each patient and assign her/him a visit (or not). They had to manage the limited resources available (time in particular) and establish priorities. Because there were no time slots available for all, nurses had to decide. That is, to deny or delay care to some of them. As one of the participants in the research said, they 'must know how to ask the right questions and read between the lines all the time'. However, it took more than intuition: the allocation process was guided and aided by a computer system that gave access to the time schedule and where all patients' data was stored and checked. Information at disposal in the system included:

- The patient's name, national registration number, and address
- List of visits to the health care centre
- List of prescribed drugs
- The doctors' patient-record
- The nurses' patient-record (VIPS[4])
- A 'note-book' for communication and messaging
- Access to an intranet with e-mail, information about access to other health care providers, interpreters services etc.
- The appointment schedule

When a patient came (or called), the nurse asked for an ID so she could access the file. Looking at the file, asking questions and consulting the availability of appointments in the system the nurse had to make a decision and allocate the patient in a time slot (or not). The system had been programmed so that it divided the working time in 15 minutes slots (the duration of a normal visit). There were different kind of visits, though: A) emergency visits, B) planned visits to doctors/nurses booked by nurses, C) planned visits to doctors booked by doctors, D) doctors' prescription time (time to write prescription – with or without patients), E) administration, F) coffee and lunch. A further restriction decided by the centre was that only emergency appointments could be given for the same day. All other appointments were given in a month's time. Therefore, the nurses were confronted routinely with the decision of giving the patient an emergency appointment for that day or making her/him way thirty days. This created a number of conflicts – between patients and nurses, between medical and technological criteria, between what is thought to be needed and what can be given, etc. However, every system has its blind spots, and nurses struggled daily to find ways of reducing the distance between criteria. For example, they could ask doctors to use their 'prescription time' to see patients, or to 'open' their time slots for nurses' bookings.

[4] VIPS is an acronym for well-being, integrity, prevention and safety, developed by Swedish nurses and used by Swedish nurses, and can also be regarded as a method for standardization.

The importance of the VIPS system went nevertheless far beyond the sorting of patients and the scheduling of visits. First, it created a comprehensive structure of information codification, storing and circulation. Secondly, it made that information accountable, both in terms of work responsibility and economic terms. The standardization of documentation was extremely important, for it allowed an easier and more precise communication among professionals, including a better transmission of the patient's record. At the same time, it made nurses exchangeable. Standardization made it irrelevant who filled in the documentation, since every nurse was supposed to comply with the set of rules. The continuity and circulation of information was not dependent upon individuals anymore, but on the system and its procedures.

> We documented earlier too, we wrote a lot: everything we made with the patients, reports to the nurse on night duty, what had happened to the patients... But it was rather arbitrary, with our own words. The documentation became more precise [when the VIPS system was implemented], so that it could be used internationally in a report, so we all knew what we referred to when we used a word. And that is very good. It's a part of the education today, the nurse education. Learning how to do the documentation. It is very well developed in comparison to the sixties or seventies when we wrote by hand, stories. The problem was that we didn't know if we were referring to the same thing. It's strange, but it worked, it turned out well. No one can say that things happened because of careless documentation. [...] Many of the questions concerning [professional] responsibility are related to insufficient documentation. There's no time for documentation. But I think it is important, I try to teach my students how to do the documentation. And not because you must protect yourself but because it's important for the patient and for medical security. (Swedish nurse 1)

The VIPS system therefore had a great impact in the organization of documentation. But as we said earlier, standardization and accountability went hand by hand in this case. And as the nurse said above, not only because a registry was produced for every action (so there's always the possibility of tracing the person responsible for it), but because the system was directly linked to financing and economic assessment. This connection needs to be described with some detail.

Every visit was referred in the computer system as a 'stick', which was the unit used for accountability and payback. All treatments had to be 'purchased' by the region, so nothing could be done without a 'stick'. Every appointment gave the centre a certain amount of money back, up to an established limit. If there were fewer visits, they got less money back. But if there were more visits they did not get that extra reimbursement back. This economically-driven design created a conflict with some of the goals of the Centre, notably health promotion. Since they could not carry on any activity without a 'stick', there was little room for it. Nurses complained this closed system had obliged them to give up one of the so-called rationales behind primary health care.

> The purchasing is so limited, and the resources are so limited, that we have to give up health promotion. The primary health care nurses from this city district meet once a month and we discuss how to increase this aspect. As it is now we integrate health promotion in almost all our meetings with patients. But the patients are already ill when they see us. We want to turn it in another direction, and meet the problem outside the health care centre, so to say: health promoting activities, community information, etc. (Swedish nurse 3)

Nurses' performance was also measured in terms of 'availability'. The criterion was that all patients should get an appointment for the same day if in emergency and all calls to the centre should be answered. Here again, the software the centre used to manage calls, TeleQ, turned into an accountability device[5]. The program not only automatically distributed the work load among operators, it also registered various indicators of performance (such as the duration of the call), that were later used to assess the 'quality' of the phone service. As one of the participants said: 'the program tells me which number to call, or which messages I should listen to... And there we sit, chained'. The following exchange during a focus group sheds some more light on the nurses' perspective on TeleQ:

> When I started to work in the primary health care the district nurse could see patients rather freely but now we have to adjust to appointment times and give service on the telephone. We have to be available for the health care centre in a different way. And this is not why I got my education, to give service calls for a health care centre. It was the preventive work that attracted me. (Swedish nurse 4)

> To fulfil your goals, this is all that counts [...] You must do a certain number of sticks every year. A diabetes patient takes one hour, that's one stick for that hour. You can carry out three injections in an hour, which equals three sticks. But there's no differentiation: one stick per treatment [regardless of the time it takes]. (Swedish nurse 5)

[5] 'TeleQ makes it possible to have telephone lines open 24 hours a day. The callers get notified when they can expect to be called back. The TeleQ users can easily set the hours for incoming and outgoing calls according to their schedule. TeleQ levels the traffic peaks and valleys thus the burden of work is evenly allocated over the working hours... The telephones become silent and the work environment becomes less stressful. The user can finish the ongoing call without experiencing the stress caused by knowing there is someone waiting on the phone before he or she takes the next call. The picture of all incoming calls on the screen creates a clear image of the working situation. The operator takes the initiative in the conversation that makes it easier to handle the call more efficiently. No customers get neglected when everybody gets through and the technique lets the employees focus on the actual communication. No one has to wait on the telephone anymore. TeleQ can be integrated with tools for analysis that helps the operator to achieve optimal capacity and facilitates work evaluations.' (Taken from their website: www.tidax.com/teleq.htm. [Accessed February 5, 2008].

Our Swedish case study graphically shows the multilayered impact of certain management software in nurses' everyday work. In a context where they enjoy a great deal of professional autonomy, these devices have however introduced the financial dimension into the daily procedures tying nurses to agreements over which they have little or no saying. No treatment or intervention outside those agreements can be practised. The number of patients and visits must be in tune with the economic aims. Medical criteria, particularly health promotion, become secondary. Nurses are confronted with a new position in their field: this economically-driven management has turned them into intermediaries between the system's efficiency and the users' demands. Nurses control the access to health care. They have become 'gate keepers'.[6]

THE LIMITS TO PROFESSIONALIZATION

New management has been frequently associated with decentralization of decision-making processes, the flattening of hierarchies and a bottom-up approach to organization, in short, with the empowerment of employees. These associations have also been widely discussed (Ackroyd et al. 2007; Bolton 2004; Hoggett 1991, 1996). The English case study illustrates how the flattening of hierarchies between nurses and doctors and the increase in work autonomy by nurses is accompanied by parallel trends of deteriorating working conditions. The English case (Norrie and Goodson 2007) demonstrates very convincingly the logic by which increase in autonomy and loss of control of working conditions are two sides of the same coin.

The upgrading of education for nurses to university level and the grounding of their knowledge in the positivist scientific paradigm provided a decisive step to gain of autonomy in relation to doctors. The hospital-based nursing colleges in England were amalgamated into the university system over the 1990s and the old emphasis in practical skills was dropped in favour of more academic disciplines like psychology and sociology (Bradshaw 2001). This in turn flattened certain areas of professional hierarchy where different professional expertise of doctors and nurses co-exist. This trend is also reflected to different degrees in the survey, where 38% of the Irish, 54% of the Finnish and 62% of the Swedish nurses agreed that there were less hierarchies nowadays than in the past (Sohlberg et al. 2007, 152). The same trend was described for the relations between nurses. The rigid and authoritative relations of the past have been superseded by rather colloquial relations among more specialized nursing roles. Teamwork is also a common practice across the cases (see also Sohlberg et al. 2007, 148, 162). Tellingly, an English nurse recalled the strict old standards in terms of dress, hygiene and rigid procedures for patient care, monitored by sister nurses.

[6] It is important to note that a similar software package was in use in Finland with very different outcomes. First, not being linked to the financing of the health system, it was seen more as a tool for organizing everyday work than as a mechanism of control. Secondly, nurses' greater degree of participation in management tended to prevent seeing such devices as mere impositions.

Older nurses supervised her work and represented a source of authority: 'I hardly ever spoke to any sister, you just wouldn't. If you did speak to hear it was only a question. [...] There was more sort of a hierarchy as such' (English nurse 1).

The process of professionalization, grounded in evidence-based practice and academic knowledge, left many of these traditional hierarchical configurations behind. A sphere of autonomy and responsibility was carved out – many times in relation to doctors. However, nurses' work has also been increasingly conditioned by external factors: economic targets, limited resources, management decisions, etc. Their newly won autonomy in terms of *doing* is thus constrained by decisions taken beyond their sphere of influence. Nurses manage everyday nursing and caring tasks, but they don't have administrative or managerial authority to alter the very framework within which they make their decisions.

The mismatch between autonomy over nursing tasks but not over the resources to execute them put additional strain on nurses. Nurses worked with an increasing number of health care assistants (HCAs) in England. HCAs carried tasks previously assigned to nurses (e.g. bathing patients, maintaining stock in pharmaceutics and instruments, taking and recording blood pressure), but they didn't take the responsibility of them. Nurses could delegate certain tasks to their HCAs, but the responsibility remained theirs. As an early-career nurse stated:

> [...] it is a dangerous way to go really [...], you do have to be careful because you are responsible for them. So ultimately it will be your fault. You have to watch your back a bit. It's your registration that is on the line if something goes wrong and that's the bottom line. I know if I make a mistake I can take the blame for that but if you are taking the blame for someone else's mistake then that is frightening. You feel a bit paranoid. (English nurse 6)

Along the same lines, the outsourcing and privatization of certain tasks such as the distribution of food or the cleaning of the wards had curtailed their sense of autonomy. As a professional group nurses ideally have the authority to decide the most adequate care for their patients. True autonomy in this sense would imply not only the ability to choose the most adequate practices but also having the resources to execute them. However, outsourcing according to cost-efficiency criteria runs precisely counter to this ideal of holistic autonomy. As one of the English nurses complained: 'The wards are shitty, the cleaners don't give a monkey's – and I wouldn't give a monkey's at four pounds money an hour either. You know, I wouldn't care that it wasn't clean.' (English nurse 3)

There was no question for nurses of the importance of hygienic standards to be maintained in their wards but clearly, their capacity for executing and achieving these standards was severely constrained by outsourcing. Similarly, they were responsible for their patients' diet. However, since food was distributed by sub-contracted, medically unqualified personnel, nurses' possibility for putting their knowledge and guidelines into practice became quite difficult.

In summary, although nurses had gained in autonomy in various respects, new methods of monitoring their work put this freedom under a tight regime of control and regulation. They had to respond to criteria of performativity and efficiency dictated by management. Their work was no longer under direct supervision by doctors or senior nurses, rather nurses had come to monitor themselves by evidencing compliance with financial targets and/or quality guidelines. As several of the interviewed nurses claimed, accountability as such is not understood as negative; it has clearly allowed raising the standards and quality of care. The crucial problem was their lack of resources, that is, the lack of autonomy to manage the temporal and economic resources necessary to meet the demanded standards.

This split between the autonomy of work and the lack of influence in changing the conditions of working is also evident from the survey. With minor differences across countries, two thirds of nurses in Ireland, Finland and Sweden stated that they didn't participate in decisions concerning the distribution of funds, staffing, or services delivered by their organization (Sohlberg et al. 2007, 195ff.). Sometimes nurses were confronted with having to decide to whom care was denied when resources were scarce. A larger quote from a nurse in England makes clearer the double constraint played by documentation guidelines and lack of resources:

> I'm the wound care link nurse here and it's frustrating to be that, because, you know, there's only so much pushing you can do for people to fill in the forms. We got an assessment policy and people don't think, you know, people assume it isn't our problem because they're going to move on from us in twelve hours, they're going to, and actually we haven't got the dressings, I mean, it's, there's nothing more disheartening that filling out a wound care assessment after you've dressed the dressing with what you know isn't the correct dressing, but because we haven't got the correct dressing, no-one will give us the correct dressing, and we can't order the correct dressing because they're going to be gone by the time it arrives. (English nurse 1)

COLLECTIVE RESPONSIBILITY

The case study in a public Finnish health care centre[7] (Kosonen and Houtsonen 2007) is an interesting counterexample of many of the previous dynamics as well as an important illustration of the transformation of the mechanics of control related to new management architectures.

First, decision-making have been increasingly decentralized from the national to the local level. Secondly, the Municipal Board of Social Welfare and Health Care implemented a number of policies aimed at redistributing authority. Administration

[7] The study was based in a primary health care centre, publicly owned and run by the municipality. The centre was located in a peripheral town, with lower standards of living than the country's average but an educational, commercial and cultural centre for the region nonetheless. All the collaborators in this study where so called consulting nurses with their reception .

and management were increasingly brought down to the health centres themselves and shared between their professionals. In the case study, there were formal monthly meetings in which decisions concerning the centre were taken. There were also less formal meetings in which everyday decisions were taken (medical supplies to be ordered, vacation days, change of patients, etc.). Decisions regarding control, supervision, planning, evaluation and documentation of nurses' work were made in monthly meetings with all the nurses, health centre assistants and the departmental head nurse. The daily tasks were planned, organised, and distributed among colleagues and then carried out independently by them. There was a great deal of mutual trust between professionals. Self-control and self-responsibility seemed to be the cornerstones of this regime of professional co-operation. When asked about this, nurses agreed upon a common sense of collaboration. As one of the participants in the study said:

> They do listen to the nurses, too, and their opinions are taken into consideration, so I feel that the decisions are taken together. We nurses are important in delivering information to the upper level, reporting what goes on here in practise, relaying the constant feedback from the patients. They do listen to us, and try to make the decisions on the basis of the feedback the patients give us as well, yes. (Finnish nurse 1)

In relation to this, management was not seen as monitoring and controlling. The organization of the unit was based on mutual trust and self-responsibility. In fact, supervisors were not present on a daily basis.

> [O]f course management monitors us, but it doesn't mean that there's someone standing behind our back all the time, the head nurse or someone. We're quite, you know, they trust us; I'd say that, that's how I see it. (Finnish nurse 2)

> Here it's mostly up to you. I mean, there's nobody to watch the way I treat the client who comes here. So you've got a big responsibility. Of course the clients may complain then, and we do get supervision or control from our supervisors. So it's very much about you yourself being sure that you know this thing, and you're saying the right thing to the client. You need to be sharp with yourself. (Finnish nurse 3)

Our fieldwork shows nurses indeed worked most of the time independently: they attended patients according to the schedule of the day, prepared treatments, documented the visits, consulted laboratory results, etc. They occasionally assisted other nurses or doctors in more complex treatments and got together with colleagues for planning and organizing. In this Finnish health centre, autonomy had been gained both in terms of *doing* and *governing* – which in turn implied that control was above all self-control. There was a common understanding of autonomy as self-responsibility, in part reaffirmed by the transfer of duties from doctors to nurses[8]. The wide recognition of professional autonomy was therefore linked to a consequent reliance on professional collective responsibility. In fact, patients and their potential complaints were probably the main mechanisms of performance monitoring, which resulted in a scrupulous practice of documentation by nurses. Once more, the response to the threat was based on self-discipline and professional confidence.

RESISTANCES, INDIFFERENCES, INFORMALITIES

We observed a somewhat convergent dynamic in the case studies based in Portugal[9], Spain[10] and Greece[11]: many of the management policies were 'filtered' by professionals in such a way that they were hardly recognizable (Pereira 2007; Safiliou-Rothschild 2007; Müller et al. 2007). Our last section is precisely dedicated to the ways management policies are interpreted, transformed, subverted, disregarded, etc. in everyday work situations. Somehow, we would like this section to be regarded as the recognition of an inevitable distance between discourses of transformation and practices of transformation. What the case studies in southern Europe show is the magnitude that this gap can reach[12]. This, in turn, raises the question of the limits of change as it is envisioned and planned from above.

[8] It is worth noting that as a consequence of the shortage of doctors, nurses had been given new tasks on the grounds of more flexible and effective caring by means of the National Treatment Guarantee Act. So there were nurses working in teams with doctors and also 'consulting' nurses that had their own offices where they worked independently.

[9] The Portuguese case study was carried in a medium sized (352 beds) public hospital. It depended on the Portuguese State and the Health Ministry ran it, though it was part of a group of hospitals with the status of a private limited enterprise with 100% public capital. They were called EPE (public business entities). This scheme allowed each entity to manage its workers with more flexibility (i.e. not based in the civil servant status), although in the particular hospital we studied the structure had remained pretty much the same. The hospital was committed, besides the obvious clinical aims, to education and research. It had its own research centre and collaborated with universities in the education of professionals.

[10] The Spanish case study was based in a medium (418 beds) hospital in Barcelona, self-defined as the avant-garde of private sector management of public health services. The Hospital belonged and was managed by a local public enterprise that emphasized commitment of professionals, continuing education and professional career. Although during our study we heard more than once that the administration of the hospital was quite remote to the daily concerns of nurses, the Hospital is indeed, as one can read in its corporate brochures, 'ten years ahead' the rest in terms of flexibility, decentralization and internal competition. It should also be noted that although we speak of the 'Spanish' case study, the results presented are not representative for the national situation. Currently there are 17 autonomous regions in Spain; administration of public health is distributed between the central Government in Madrid and those regions. When we therefore speak of the 'Spanish', this rather refers to the national identities within the Profknow Consortium than the empirical situation on the ground.

[11] The Greek case study was based in a small (160 beds) university hospital in Athens. It belonged to the Medical School of Athens University, but also received substantial donations from private donors.

[12] It should be noted that the three case studies were based in hospitals, which makes the comparison with the kind of dynamics observed in primary health centres particularly difficult, if not totally inappropriate.

As we have already seen, increasing computerization and evaluation are important components of new management strategies. These were measures certainly introduced in the hospital we studied in Greece, whose managers were proud to claim it was the only fully computerized hospital in the country. Observations, however, showed a rather limited implementation of ICT in everyday work. In fact, all the patient's documentation was filled by hand in what supposed an extremely time-consuming task for nurses (between one and two hours every day). The amount of information kept (reports of condition, tests results, treatments, reactions, etc.) created a massive problem of storage. It was only possible to have at hand the clinical history of the last 15 days – the rest filed and stored and therefore not immediately available.

This situation was explained by younger nurses as the result of a generational gap in respect to technology. They expressed their discomfort with the situation and, contrary to the official explanation, blamed it on the older professional's resistance to technology, not the lack of resources. They considered computers would accelerate the process of documentation (and free them from the boredom of repetition) and save useful time in a context of nurses shortage. Finally, it would be better for the treatment of patients, since their complete file would be easily accessible. As one male nurse participating in the study put it:

> I have a computer at home and I am a skilful user but I am pessimistic about the future of computerization in the hospital. I feel that the older generation has a different mentality, they are negative and they cannot accept computerization. I am afraid that, if computerization would become the rule in the hospital, only the men and only 1-2 young women would follow. (Greek nurse 3)

As for evaluation measures, professionals showed extreme mistrust and cynicism about attempts to introduce external evaluation. Not only were they regarded as inappropriate, they were readily deactivated by professionals: existing evaluation forms had not been passed for years – and when so they had been made unusable by giving maximum marks in all questions.

A very interesting area of reform and negotiation in Spain, Greece and Portugal was the reconfiguration of professional responsibilities. In line with the general trend, there has been a continuous process of professionalization of nurses. This process has usually been linked to the redistribution of authority, particularly between doctors and nurses. In Spain these attempts took the form of the 'team of professionals', introduced during the comprehensive reform of the public health sector carried in the nineties. It was directed at overcoming the traditional hierarchy between doctors and the rest of professionals by introducing more horizontal teams where all professional should work together. About ten years after its introduction, we found little evidence of them in our observations of daily work. The everyday 'team' seemed to be restricted to nurses and nurse assistants. In fact, in some areas the relation with the doctors was quite limited. In the post-operation unit we observed they rarely met, even though theoretically they form part of the same work team. Their paths crossed in the corridor, but they never visited a patient together. They neither took breaks together nor did the doctors enter the nurses' meeting room. In fact, nurses' breaks systematically coincided in time with doctors' visits, making encounters highly improbable. In the words of one the nurses 'they mind their business and we ours' – but cordially.

In the Greek hospital, the restructuring of the division of labour faced contextual imperatives. On the one hand, the shortage of nurses pushed nursing assistants to carry some of their tasks. At the same time, doctors delegated some of their tasks to nurses – the ones they defined as 'unimportant' and 'time-consuming', without recognition or legal coverage. This resulted in a controversial perception of autonomy – even if observations in the hospital showed a rather fluent stream of collaboration between professional.

> I feel that the profession of nursing is not an independent profession. Nurses depend from doctors; they always need doctors' orders and because of this there is sometimes considerable conflict and contention. Nurses often perform treatments because the doctor does not feel like bothering with them but formally the medical profession doesn't agree to classify these activities as nurses' actions. (Greek nurse 1)

> I don't feel that I have autonomy but I would not want to have more autonomy because it would be too much responsibility. As things are, the doctor can cover me and I can cover the doctor. (Greek nurse 2)

> Yes I have considerable autonomy in decision–making in my job. I take orders for the quantity and type of blood that is needed. But then, I in collaboration with my colleagues can manage everything; we handle existing problems and have a certain degree of responsibility and power. If, for example, too much blood is needed but the supply is limited, we suggest to the surgeons to postpone surgeries that are not urgent. Of course, there is also a supervisor and a director who is a physician blood specialist with whom I discuss when there are problems and she is the one who takes the final decision. (Greek nurse 3)

In Portugal, the autonomy of the nursing profession is recognized by law, which literally says that "nurses' practice is complementary to that of the other health professionals, but sharing the same level of dignity and professional autonomy" (REPE 1996: art. 8). Observations showed nurses to be in fact quite independent: nurses in charge of each specific area were responsible for work schedules, evaluation of care needs, distribution of personal, managing of auxiliary staff and basic logistics. Once priorities were set and tasks distributed, nurses carried on their practice rather autonomously. When working with doctors, however, the equality stated above was rather contingent. In all of the three services observed, there were very different dynamics and arrangements.

> We get on very well but no one interferes with the others' job. But we get on very well, perfectly, nurses, technicians, doctors, perfectly, but no one interferes with the work of the others. (Portuguese nurse 1)

> Nurses are not very autonomous in here, I think they aren't. [...] The service chief and the director [both doctors] are the ones who establish the proceedings. [...] So, we play our [secondary] part and try to do our best, but there really is very little autonomy in this service. (Portuguese nurse 2)

We encountered a particular combination of informal arrangements to be prevalent, while not specifically sanctioned and always mediated by the remains of old formalities in the relation with other professionals, especially doctors. In all the three cases there was a significant tendency to informal processes of self-organization among nurses. By informal we mean dynamics that were not related to any official policy or directive. Sometimes they were at odds with them. Other times, these 'informalities' were just an adaptation of the rules.

In the Portuguese hospital we studied, slight adaptations of rules helped smoothing the functioning of the centre. Nurses, for example, were according to the established procedures assigned to particular patients. They were supposed to take care of them exclusively. In practice, however, nurses cooperated and helped each other, making the distribution of tasks much more flexible and shared. In addition, due to the work-shifts nature of hospital work, communication between nurses was extremely important. Interestingly, key information transmission took place informally in shared open spaces. In a similar fashion, in-service learning was a rather informal process in which the 'experienced' shared their knowledge with the 'newcomers'. What interests us here is how an informal process of competence recognition among peers (basically through demonstration in the work place) turned into an established dynamic among them. Regardless of the official one-month supervision, 'older colleagues' further extended their training and performance control tasks. 'There's always an older colleague to help you' was a recurrent motto when talking about this.

The Spanish hospital showed a similar pattern in this respect. Transmission of information happened in an open, often unpredictable way (at coffee breaks, in the corridors, etc.). Likewise, evaluation and control was mainly enforced informally by peers. In this sense, it is relevant to consider that nurses worked pretty much autonomously and without any other supervision than themselves. They had their recognized areas of knowledge and fields of action. It depended on the will, self-esteem and self-confidence of each nurse the way it was played out. This autonomy could include the interpretation of patient behaviour in relation to medication, making arrangements for commissioning a medical analysis – which had to be signed by a doctor – or even refusing to proceed with a treatment when in disagreement[13]. In fact, the supervisor nurse (one for each unit) rarely interceded in daily work. Decisions regarding shifts, vacations and other

[13] One of the participants gave us an example of this when she refused a doctor's request to further treat a coma patient. In her opinion, the moment had come where disconnecting this patient should be seriously considered. Although the doctor got furious, she maintained her position and professional ethics. She was unsure what would have happened if another nurse wouldn't have done the job. But the fact that there were no consequences for her whatsoever shows that her professional autonomy and capacity of decision taking has a wide and not so clearly defined reserve.

organization issues were normally taken by the nurses themselves (balancing seniority, special needs, etc.) and then signed by the supervisor.

It is important to point at the way this informal quality of relations is in itself a form of (peer) control. It is precisely through the *de facto* autonomy that nurses have in their everyday duties that this form of regulation becomes essential. It's not the managers, or the doctors, the authority that rule the units. They can (and do) set some procedures, but what happens within them is far from those formalities. At the same time, this kind of autonomy in *doing* and even in aspects of *governing* is nowhere sanctioned or recognized, and therefore remains contingent, precarious, outside professional achievements.

CONCLUDING REMARKS

In this chapter we have attempted to contribute to the debate around the impact of NPM in nurses' work life by looking at more or less detailed evidence. We read across the seven national reports and selected those themes we found more pertinent to the discussion. Our main argument is that NPM has indeed reshaped many aspects of nurses' everyday work and has resulted, in combination with other processes such as professionalization, in a simultaneous (and non paradoxical) increase in autonomy and control. We haven't attempted, though, to draw a homogeneous map. We have tried to retain the specificity of the data gathered and point at those non-convergent dynamics. This, we hope, could contribute to a more complex and pondered understanding of the effects of new management schemes. Our case studies show how similar policies have produced dissimilar results in different contexts. For example, the great impact accountability has created in working conditions in England or Ireland are in sharp contrast with the loose dynamics observed in the Southern States. Also, the level of self-management that Finnish nurses enjoy greatly differs from that of their colleagues in Sweden – even if similar procedures have been introduced.

As stated above, we have been primarily concerned with presenting evidence of the different meanings NPM has adopted in the countries studied. We showed how the pressure of cost-control is shaping nurses' daily work in England, Ireland and Sweden. These three cases were important in illustrating how economic and health care goals are related and interfered. The Finnish case was presented as a kind of counterexample, in which self-control and collective responsibility prevailed over discipline in management. It was a strong case for professionalization of nurses. Lastly, Portugal, Greece and Spain offered interesting evidence of the limits of restructuring policies as they are negotiated in practice. Nurses here demonstrated powerful agency that, ranging from cynicism to resistance, managed to reshape the impulse of reform.

This heterogeneity poses a key question: how can such wide differences be explained? What are the components and the agents that account for it? Here we must be cautious: the factors involved are so varied and our understanding of the processes so incipient that we can only raise it as a question for further research. Nevertheless, our project constitutes a first step towards appreciating the recent restructuring of health care throughout Europe.

REFERENCES

Ackroyd, S., Kirkpatrick. I. & Walker, R. M. (2007). Public Management Reform in the UK and Its Consequences for Professional Organization: A Comparative Analysis. *Public Administration*, 85(1), 9-26.

Bolton, S. C. (2004). A Simple Matter of Control? NHS Hospital Nurses and New Management. *Journal of Management Studies*, 41(2), 317-333.

Bradshaw, A. (2001). *The project 2000 Nurse:* The Remaking of British General Nursing, 1978-2000. London: Whurr.

Dupont, M. & Sugrue, C. (2007) Irish Nurses' Work and Life Under Restructuring: Professional Experiences, Knowledge and Expertise in Changing Contexts. In T. Kosonen & Houtsonen, J. (eds) *European Nurses' Life and Work Under Restructuring: Professional Experiences, Knowledge and Expertise in Changing Contexts*. Deliverable 5 in the EU sixth framework project Professional Knowledge in Education and Health: Restructuring work and life between the State and the citizens in Europe. http://profknow.net/files/results/D05_European_Nurses_Life_and_Work_under_Restructuring.pdf [Accessed July 2008]

Harlow, C. (2002). *Accountability in the European Union*. Oxford: Oxford University Press

Hoggett, P. (1991). A New Management in the Public Sector? *Policy & Politics*, 19(4), 243-256.

Hoggett, P. (1996). New Modes of Control in the Public Services'. *Public Administration*, 74(1), 9-32.

Kosonen, T. & Houtsonen, J. (2007) Finnish Nurses. In T. Kosonen & Houtsonen, J. (eds) *European Nurses' Life and Work Under Restructuring: Professional Experiences, Knowledge and Expertise in Changing Contexts*. Deliverable 5 in the EU sixth framework project Professional Knowledge in Education and Health: Restructuring work and life between the State and the citizens in Europe. http://profknow.net/files/results/D05_European_Nurses_Life_and_Work_under_Restructuring.pdf [Accessed July 2008]

Müller, J., Larrain, V., Creus, A., Marrero, I., Muntadas, M., Hernández, F. & Sancho, J. M. (2007) Case Study Report: Life Histories – Nurses Spain. In T. Kosonen & Houtsonen, J. (eds) *European Nurses' Life and Work Under Restructuring: Professional Experiences, Knowledge and Expertise in Changing Contexts*. Deliverable 5 in the EU sixth framework project Professional Knowledge in Education and Health: Restructuring work and life between the State and the citizens in Europe. http://profknow.net/files/results/D05_European_Nurses_Life_and_Work_under_Restructuring.pdf [Accessed July 2008]

Norrie, C. & Goodson, I. (2007) English Nurses' Work and Life Under Restructuring: Professional Experiences Knowledge and Expertise in Changing Contexts. In T. Kosonen & Houtsonen, J. (eds) *European Nurses' Life and Work Under Restructuring: Professional Experiences, Knowledge and Expertise in Changing Contexts*. Deliverable 5 in the EU sixth framework project Professional Knowledge in Education and Health: Restructuring work and life between the State and the citizens in Europe. http://profknow.net/files/results/D05_European_Nurses_Life_and_Work_under_Restructuring.pdf [Accessed July 2008]

Pollitt, C. & Bouckaert, G. (2005). *Public Management Reform. A Comparative Analysis*. Oxford: Oxford University Press

Pollitt, C., Birchall, J. & Putman, K. (1998). *Decentralising Public Service Management*. London: Macmillan.

Pereira, H. (2007) Portuguese Nurses' Lives Under Restructuring - Case Study Report. In T. Kosonen & Houtsonen, J. (eds) *European Nurses' Life and Work Under Restructuring: Professional Experiences, Knowledge and Expertise in Changing Contexts*. Deliverable 5 in the EU sixth framework project Professional Knowledge in Education and Health: Restructuring work and life between the State and the citizens in Europe. http://profknow.net/files/results/D05_European_Nurses_Life_and_Work_under_Restructuring.pdf [Accessed July 2008]

Safiliou-Rothschild, C. (2007) Greek Nurses' Work and Life Under Restructuring: Professional Experiences, Knowledge and Expertise in Changing Contexts. In T. Kosonen & Houtsonen, J. (eds) *European Nurses' Life and Work Under Restructuring: Professional Experiences, Knowledge and Expertise in Changing Contexts*. Deliverable 5 in the EU sixth framework project Professional Knowledge in Education and Health: Restructuring work and life between the State and the citizens in Europe. http://profknow.net/files/results/D05_European_Nurses_Life_and_Work_under_Restructuring.pdf [Accessed July 2008]

Sohlberg, P., Czaplicka, M., Lindblad, S., Houtsonen, J., Müller, J., Morgan, G., Wärvik, M., Dupont, M., Norrie, C., Kitching, K., Kosonen, T. (2007). *Professional Expertise under Restructuring: Comparative Studies of Education and Health Care. The Survey Study.* Deliverable 3 in the EU sixth framework project Professional Knowledge in Education and Health: Restructuring work and life between the State and the citizens in Europe. http://www.profknow.net/files/results/WP3_Final_report.pdf [Accessed January 2008].

Wärvik, G-B. (2007) Nurses' Life Histories: The Swedish Case. In T. Kosonen & Houtsonen, J. (eds) *European Nurses' Life and Work Under Restructuring: Professional Experiences, Knowledge and Expertise in Changing Contexts.* Deliverable 5 in the EU sixth framework project Professional Knowledge in Education and Health: Restructuring work and life between the State and the citizens in Europe. http://profknow.net/files/results/D05_European_Nurses_Life_and_Work_under_Restructuring.pdf [Accessed July 2008]

HELDER ROCHA PEREIRA & CONSTANTINA SAFILIOU-ROTHSCHILD

EMERGING WORK TRANSITIONS IN THE NURSING PROFESSION

INTRODUCTION

Since the mid 1980s, many professions, including nursing, have experienced significant transitions in work specifications. These transitions have come about mainly because of *restructuring* that may be understood as a global movement set in a neo-liberal approach, the main concepts of which are decentralization, deregulation, privatization and *marketization* (Beach 2005). It may also be understood in a stricter sense as related to political changes that have taken place in areas and activities traditionally associated with the welfare state (Goodson & Norrie 2005). Some of these work transitions introduced into public services emphasized the justification for all actions to be based upon the need to make services economically more efficient, instead of promoting professional judgement about the best practice to follow. These transitions have affected to a considerable extent the way nurses perform activities such as how they relate to patients, how they define themselves in the organizational context and, finally, the way they adjust their professional lifestyle within this new context.

While these work transitions emerge in different ways in the different countries studied, nurses see the overall evaluation of the consequences of these transitions as negative for work performance. The experiences of nurses who participated in the study indicate two factors with a strong impact on European nurses' life and work (Houtsonen et al. 2007). First, there is the problem of shortage of time available for nursing care, driven by tightening efficiency concerns and restructuring policies. This is due to shortage of staff, lack of resources, nurses' new roles and administrative demands for documentation. These conditions contribute to the increase of nurses' workload and stress, problems in work-life balance and, in some cases, lower work morale. Due to shortage of time, nurses feel more and more difficulties in managing the administration of proper patient care according to their professional ideals. It also contributes to the inability to apply knowledge that is regarded as central according to professional standards (Kosonen & Houtsonen 2007b). Secondly, recruitment and employment contract criteria have become tighter in several contexts, causing trouble especially to young and novice nurses. This opens the discussion as to how working conditions affect both professional practice and personal life. Issues as shortage, decrease of time available for nursing care, low morale, low salaries and, in some countries, changes in labour security must also be addressed in terms of their impact on patients' quality and safety of care.

J. Houtsonen, G.-B. Wärvik (Eds.), European Nurses' Life and Work Under Restructuring pp. 95-116.

There is, however, another type of restructuring that has taken place in the nursing profession, at least in the two countries for which there are relevant data, the consequences of which for work performance and the status of the nursing profession are seen as positive. This is the restructuring resulting from men's entry into the previously women's profession of nursing. Although this restructuring is not directly related to government reforms and politics, it is bringing important changes to the nursing profession, some of them not yet felt.

While it is common for government reforms to be seen as very distant from workers' (in this case nurses') daily concerns and life, in this particular chapter, besides identifying the structural measures that have taken place, we shall examine nurses' experience of impacts, as expressed by them in interviews. In this way, a more complete understanding of restructuring processes may be achieved. Based on data collected from different national studies (Kosonen & Houtsonen 2007b), we shall try to understand to what extent political, institutional and structural changes are viewed as significant and how these changes are adapted in nurses' professionals' working lives.

NURSES' EXPERIENCES OF RESTRUCTURING: CONTEXT AND IMPACT ON PROFESSIONAL PRACTICE

Focusing on the field of healthcare and taking into account the way that neo-liberal management measures, aiming at cost accounting, optimisation of resources, decrease of expenses and balance of public service's accounts, have influenced different contexts of public health care (Beach 2005), it is important to reflect upon some issues such as: How do the changes take place from nurses' perspective? How do nurses' actions vary as a consequence of changes in working conditions? Which particular changes in nurses' working conditions have more direct impact on their actions? How do changes in management, which are necessary for the balancing of resources, relate with the possibility of performing a truly professional role?

Holistic Care and Curing

There is considerable tension around what is considered the *core* of nursing as a profession, as a distinct way of being among health care professions and the inability to put that *core* to practice. This discussion is important because care has been considered the essential focus for nursing as a profession and it is characterised by a global approach to patients, centred on the evaluation of their needs in a holistic perspective – as many nurses never cease to reinforce. Cody (2000) considers that nursing has walked a long path that has shifted the emphasis from the cure to the co-participation of nurses and patients in the development of quality of life according to patients' perspective. Thus is born the concept of patient advocacy, which implies that the nurse's loyalty goes primarily to the patient, a concept that can create dilemmas and confrontation within the health care team as well as in the context of health organizations.

The provision of holistic health care requires time to establish a relation with the patient, time for assessment, decision-making and action. Such an approach distances itself from a practice based manly in actions of technical nature, measured by the time that it takes and the number of tasks performed. This theme is not of little importance because it is imbued in what has been ideally considered as the scope of nursing performance, at the same level as professional autonomy and nursing knowledge. This discussion is frequently set around the care *versus* cure dichotomy. In the former case, one must approach the global needs of patients, providing them with physical comfort, spiritual, emotional and social care, an approach claimed by most nurses as their scope of action. The later is more oriented toward cure that is toward the technique, an approach closer to the medical profession. This type of dichotomy is considered by many as a wasted discussion, since there is no care without taking into account cure and, at the same time, one does not expect a cure without being concerned with care (Kottow 2001).[1]

Here it is important to note that the great emphasis on care of patients in a holistic manner may not be so accentuated by male nurses. As Safiliou-Rothschild (2007) writes, because according to male stereotypes men are expected to be rational and scientific (rather than nurturing), male nurses may lean more toward the curing dimension. This holds true for Konstantinos, the Greek male nurse who appreciates the specialized, technological, scientific aspects of his work more than the direct contact with sick people:

> When I started working in the university hospital, I discovered laboratory work and research and decided that that is what suits me best. Although initially that I liked most was the direct contact with patients and now although there is no direct contact with sick people, I am satisfied since there is contact with doctors, with surgical services, with the operations and with blood transfusion. In addition, I feel that it is most important that if a patient needs surgery, blood donation is at the first line. In this way, I have the satisfaction that I contribute to patients' recovery although from far away. Some patients I had never seen came to thank me and the entire unit, when they got well, a source of tremendous satisfaction that has made me love my work. (Safiliou-Rothschild 2007, 160).

Furthermore, the Greek male nurse is satisfied with his status because his work resembles research and he feels that scientific progress has helped the nursing profession to be continuously upgraded and to improve the quality of his work. Konstantinos says:

> I feel that the general conditions of nursing have improved considerably from 1989, when I started. Now there are better machines, better technology, more knowledge, many opportunities for training, many conferences and nurses are able to learn as much as they can. I feel that because of these positive changes, it is now possible to control much better the blood given to patients (Safiliou-Rothschild 2007, 161).

[1] The issues around knowledge and autonomy will be deeply discussed in the next chapters, taking into account this dichotomy.

Even if we do not consider care and cure as a dichotomy, we must recognize that nursing professionals deal with patients in a different way than physicians. In the nursing perspective, the orientation is toward the human being seen as a whole continuously interacting with dynamic, temporary, historic and cultural worlds (Chen 2000). Thus, in this perspective, the complexities and unique experiences of each patient are recognized (Chen 2000; Newman 2002). There is considerable agreement among most nurses that they value patients as whole human beings instead of restricting their interest merely to clinical conditions. This attitude sets the transition from a professional approach based on the disease and on mainly physical and technical aspects, towards a more inclusive approach in which caring does not overlook these aspects but, rather, includes them hand in hand with a wider relational, social, psychological and spiritual perspective.

These considerations are appealing since we aim to understand the impacts of restructuring measures on nurses' professional practice. We shall examine the restructuring impact on professional practice in the light of this new environment of health care giving, divided between concerns about the control of costs and the care of a gradually older population. The question centres on how working conditions offered to nurses interact with nurses playing a part they define as their appropriate role.

Shortage of Time to Care

It must be noted that the contexts in which the national studies have been developed vary considerably in terms of type of context (Hospital *versus* Health Centre), social characteristics of the patient populations and institutional resources. In addition, there are differences in the roles played by nurses in the health care system of each country, the number of male nurses practicing, as well as different degrees and qualifications required for occupying certain positions.

Notwithstanding the weight these factors represent in nurses' daily work, depending on the national context, our attention was focused upon more general aspects as the professional/personal impacts felt by the participants resulting from reorganization of national health care services. Deriving from this focus of analysis emerges the central theme throughout the different project country studies: Shortage of time to care. This is the most evident aspect that connects the different settings studied, no matter what the different specificities (refractions) of each country may

[2] However, it must be noted that the profile of the new generation of Greek nurses has been drastically changed by significant changes in terms of higher educational level, higher socio-economic status and a more 'liberated' gender profile that allows them to have fewer children and to continue their career after childbirth (Safiliou-Rothschild, 2007). These changes considerably affect their performance of their professional roles.

be.[2] The causes, the forms, the working contexts differ, but, in the midst of national differences, nurses[3] in this study reinforce this reality: the role that organizations expect of them, the lack of qualified personnel, high shift rotation, the increase of extra working hours, the lack of control over activities that once used to be supervised by them and work overload, all contributing to the shift of the professional attitude hitherto considered central for their profession toward an immediate, technical response based on giving physical care to patients.

Strategies Dealing with the Shortage of Time to Care

When considering shortage of time for care, situations of nurses understaffing and the lack of properly qualified human resources are clearly the most common situations that present constraints to ideal professional practice.

Concerning the shortage of nurses, the situation is different in each country. English nurses, for example, report a paradox. On the one hand, there is lack of nurses and deterioration of working conditions[4], but, on the other hand, their greatest fear is the risk of getting fired because of personnel release for economic reasons. The new measures that aim to control expenses in the health sector include reduction of staff in health services (nurses included). Despite the recognition of lack of nurses, positions for early-career nurses are scarce (Norrie & Goodson 2007).

This situation leads to fear of redundancy and consequently of being laid-off, which affects nurses' work organization. The fear of being laid-off affects both nurses with precarious contracts but also those who have a permanent contract, since staff release is taking place at different levels. As Maurier and Northcott (2000) had already found, when studying the effect of job uncertainty and health status during restructuring in the 1990's, the threat of being laid-off or having a co-worker laid-off has negative impacts also on those who keep their job. An increase in workload in an environment of frustration and anger results in poor health also for nurses spared of lay-off.

In the Irish case, the lack of nurses is equally a recurring theme. Changes in professional training curricula and the high rate of qualified nurses leaving the country has forced the government to take special measures in public hospitals, such as schedule flexibility and international recruitment of nurses. More flexible contract forms allow permanent work on a part-time basis and are meant to attract nurses that are not presently working to get back to public hospitals (Dupont & Sugrue 2007).

Hiring foreign nurses has been frequent. However, they are given a short adaptation time. This also implies more work for other nurses who need to do all the work for which these nurses had not been trained and, at the same time, they have to integrate and re-train on the job these foreign newcomers.

---

[3] Finnish nurses must be considered an exception to this scenario. In fact the Finnish study doesn't report serious shortage in terms of lack of staff or resources (Kosonen & Houtsonen, 2007a).

[4] Annual NHS Staff Survey reports that 74% of nurses work extra hours due the demands of the job (cit. Kosonen & Houtsonen, 2007b).

> Some of them are excellent [... they] are taking charge of the ward but they would be there... four and five years at this point. Some of them definitely wouldn't be up to that. (Nora, Irish nurse) (Dupont & Sugrue 2007, 100)

Consequently, under some circumstances, the hiring of foreign nurses has increased the workload of Irish trained nurses. Furthermore, hiring foreign nurses is something that worries international organizations because it is considered inefficient for solving present nurses' global shortage. In fact, according to data from the *International Council of Nurses*[5] (ICN, 2006), in countries such as the United Kingdom, Canada, the U.S. and Australia, the percentage of healthcare professionals trained outside the country is as high as 25%. This recruitment strategy, besides integration difficulties due to the existence of distinct cultures, worsens the lack of nurses in the countries of origin; contributes to the decrease of sustainable conditions of the healthcare systems in these countries; and raises an ethical dimension (Aiken et al. 2004). Thus, international recruitment does not seem to be an adequate solution for the problem of nurses' shortage in a global perspective.

Irish nurses talk about staff shortages, limited resources and intense workload and how this shortage impacts their work. By saying that they have to set working priorities when facing workload, once again they imply that there is a gap between the professional ideal of quality and holistic care and care provided under actual working conditions. Nora illustrates this feeling perfectly, by giving an example of her daily work. When setting priorities in her activities, she says that due to lack of time, sometimes some aspects of care such as her clients' oral hygiene are left behind: "*it's not that I don't want to do it or I don't aim to do it. It's just that I haven't got the time often and you are rushing a lot.*" (Dupont & Sugrue 2007, 99). To realize at the shift's end that there nursing tasks were not performed is a main factor facing nurses' perception about not delivering quality care. "*Low morale is caused by low staffing. It is horrible going home and thinking and knowing that you have not done your job properly and you have not looked after someone as well as you would have liked to because you haven't physically hadn't had the time to do it.*" (English nurse in Norrie & Goodson 2007, 69). Interestingly, Sochalski (2001), studying issues regarding staffing, quality of care and patient outcomes, reached the conclusion that workload increase by itself is not significant for nurses' perception of the quality of care. From nurses' perspective, it is when increased workload is combined with unfinished care that it has a pronounced influence on quality care.

An intense feeling of dissatisfaction also emerges amidst Greek nurses confronted with shortage of professionals, which has a negative impact on their work, on their access to extra training and on the quality of their work. The understaffing of nurses is due to the fact that the government does not want to increase the number of permanent public servants (that cannot be fired) and resorts to short-term contractual hiring of nurses. However, it has to be pointed out that although there is a considerable

[5] The International Council of Nurses (ICN) founded in 1899, is a federation of national nurses' associations representing nurses in 128 countries.

number of nursing jobs in the many private hospitals in Athens (and the entire country), most nurses report preferring to work in public hospitals because of job security. They correctly perceive that in private hospitals work requirements are much harder and if their performance is not satisfactory, they can get fired. However, job security in public hospitals has as negative side the discontinuous and uncertain nature of contractual work that most nurses prefer while they are waiting to become civil servants rather than accept a job in a private hospital (Safiliou-Rothschild 2007). Such short-term contracts are of course disruptive for institutional management and efficacy:

> [...] the need to hire contractual nursing personnel creates problems because by the time that they get adjusted to the work, the 8 months have passed and they have to leave. This is very difficult for the permanent personnel who and to help them adjust, have to "teach" them or at least to guide them (Maria, Greek nurse) (Safiliou-Rothschild 2007, 154).

This situation causes dissatisfaction because of increased workload (due to both the shortage of personnel and the demands of integration periods) and difficulties experienced in being able to give quality care to patients.

In Greece, the shortage of nurses is also reflected in the lack of permanent experienced nurses, who have to share their working environment with nurses, cyclically hired for medium-term contracts. The coexistence of nursing aid personnel with the lack of nurses has direct implications for task performance, making it necessary for tasks to be assigned according to needs instead according to staff qualifications. Consequently, there is no clear definition between the tasks developed by nurses and those performed by nursing aid personnel (Safiliou-Rothschild 2007).

Even though Spanish nurses do not refer directly to shortage situations, they point out experiencing lack of time to care due to the increasing demands of their working environment (Müller et al. 2007).

> [...] This is how things always are done. Lets increase, lets increase numbers and later we will talk about the additional staff and space required. And this burns you out. It burns you out because to work this way is very stressing. (Jenny, Spanish nurse) (Müller et al. 2007, 210).

Once again, they reinforce not being able to give care beyond technical aspects and complain about the constant increase of work that is asked them, without proper reward.

Gatekeeping instead of patient care

Another set of restructuring conditions brings up the shortage of resources as responsible for certain constraints among Swedish nurses. The Swedish nurses work as gatekeepers and controllers of access to health care (Wärvik 2007). Working in a health centre, they are responsible for planning patients' appointments. Because not all patients who go to the health centre for an appointment manage to get one, these nurses have to deal with that situation, by sending patients to other healthcare services or by asking them to come back another day. Despite not having brought up the shortage of nurses, in fact having to play patient gate keeping makes nurses recognize the frailty of what nurses consider to be their role, when confronted with what they are actually asked to do. On the other hand, according to the contracts of services paid by these health centres, the institution gets paid only for pre-negotiated services. In the case of this particular health centre, it is only paid for actual medical and nursing appointments. All other activities not included in this contract are no longer being accepted, because they are not seen as priorities for institutional funding. As a result of service reorganization, nurses perform activities they did not expect to perform on the basis of their professional training.

> But the district nurse is more involved with serving the doctors and answering the telephone. When I started to work in the primary health care the district nurse could see patients rather free but now we have to adjust to appointment times and give service on the telephone. Be available in a different way, for the health care centre. And this is not why I took my education, to give service to a health care centre. But it was this (the prevention work) that attracted me. /.../ They take the district nurse to the Tele Q[6] and to the waiting room work. But a district nurse should not work like that. (Swedish nurse) (Wärvik 2007, 246)

The new roles nurses must play inside the health centre, as well as the new organization set around hired services, make nurses feel constrained. They feel they can no longer use their professional free will when organizing institutional work. One of the Swedish nurses specifically refers to that aspect: "*But now we must be the police in an organisation we cannot influence, this is different. It's not about economic consciousness, because this I think is good, it's something else*" (Wärvik 2007, 251). Recognizing the costs of services, a result of restructuring, is considered positive. However, these compulsory changes have placed nurses in contradictory situations in relation to administration demands, medical doctors' and patient's requests and, once again, are responsible for nurses' difficulty to implement a professional organization in the institution (Wärvik 2007). Nurses feel cornered between patients' needs and institutional limitations, a situation that contributes to the increase of tension in the patient/nurse relation (Kosonen & Houtsonen 2007b). Such a situation seems to invert the professional ideal. Instead of being the professional who help, who consider patients' needs in a holistic way nurses often limit their actions to giving immediate and necessary care.

Increased professional workload

These new professional demands when facing restructuring processes are increasing professionals' workload. Time spent with patients is diminishing and, instead, there

[6] Tele Q is a computer based queue system that controls and orders the phone calls from patients seeking an appointment. The system allows nurses to answer telephone calls from patients (Wärvik, 2007).

is an increase of hours spent in administrative tasks (Baumann 2007), an overload that is seen by nurses as avoidable, unless if there were more personnel. In fact, the International Council of Nurses (ICN 2006) has concluded that in order for safe nursing staffing to be achieved, models developed to calculate institutional personnel needs should pay special attention to the time spent by nurses in the performance of their role, so safe staffing can be reached. According to ICN, although some models today are useful to quantify and identify nurses' tasks, in some contexts they do not reach more than 40% of the actual work performed by nurses. This is due to the fact that these programs do not take into consideration the intellectual and cognitive tasks involved in the activities performed. Irish participants constantly bring up these changes in the demands of working conditions since services are evaluated both in terms of quality and legal responsibility. Thus, even demands of written reports and all related documentation have increased. Nevertheless, all extra time spent performing these tasks is not taken into account, and, consequently, this leads to work overload. As an example, one of the Irish nurses clearly points out the effects of changes on how to deal with incidents. Before, if a client fell off a bed, he/she would once again be sent to bed, assessed and asked whether he/she wanted a cup of tea. Nowadays, there is a whole number of steps to be followed in the same situation, as Aideen illustrates: "*Documentation must be filled out, insurance people informed, risk management informed, families informed. It's all what should be happening but it's a time-consuming lengthy process*" (Dupont & Sugrue 2007, 108). Clearly, during the last years, nurses see the organizational climate as increasingly more demanding (Solberg et al. 2007).

Other important impacts of restructuring are work overload due to paper work related to the care that was given to the patient or completing documents related to the implementation of quality systems. This type of changes, along with a greater consciousness of care costs is not considered negative *per se*. However, these activities are time-consuming, a fact not well accepted by nurses when they are faced with under staffing. Writing down an exact report of the care provided can be important both for nurses' protection, when facing any legal complaints, as well as for ensuring the continuation of care giving by other professionals and as a guarantee of payment for the provided care. Nevertheless, no matter how important such documentation may be, it is time consuming.

The Greek study points out how the lack of computerization of the nursing documentation unnecessarily wastes time and accentuates existing nursing shortages, while frustrating the younger generation of nurses. This lack of computerization is mainly due to the fact that nursing supervisors, who are in their 50's, although they followed the obligatory training seminar in computers, do not know how to use computers and resist using them. In private Greek hospitals, however, computerization is widely used because business has to be efficient and profitable and cannot afford to waste nurses' time by endless recording needed information manually (Safiliou-Rothschild 2007).

New criteria for Recruitment and Employment

Another relevant factor emerging from the present study is new forms of contracting nurses. In the new context of welfare state, there is a tendency to reduce the number of civil servants giving way to decentralised forms of contracting, characterised by less stable conditions. In fact, short-term contracts and flexible schedules for work increase and precarious work is a useful term to describe the situation. By 'precarity' we refer to a set of worsening living conditions and uncertainty related with unstable working conditions (Müller et al. 2007).

This is the present situation in Portugal. In the last years, most public hospitals have adopted entrepreneurial forms of management. Even though political speeches mention the lack of nurses in the country, nurses point out that there is a boom of nursing training courses and consequently increasing availability of these professionals in the market. This situation leads to waiting periods between nurses finishing their training and actually starting to work. It also allows institutions to employ short-term recruitment strategies to deal with staff shortage.

> It's three months, they have a period of holidays, generally, they work for three months more, they reach the end of that half year term and they are fired, two days later they are hired again only and exclusively in order to get another contract, because after three contracts, we are obliged get a bond with the institution. That way, they are fired and there's no such obligation and that doesn't provide stability to anyone. (Alexandra, Portuguese nurse) (Pereira 2007, 177).

This new reality makes it more difficult for nurses to access their first job and is combined with an increase of job rotation in health institutions among newly graduated nurses during their first years of work. Furthermore, these professionals who chose nursing because it was considered a safe working choice, are presently facing difficulties in getting hired. This new context changes the power relations between young nurses and the administration boards of health institutions.

> ... are you quitting? That's okay; you don't want it? Okay. There will always be someone to replace you. (...) There are loads of nurses willing to work here. (...) This is no proper way to deal with nurses and to keep the nurses satisfied and I feel somewhat frustrated myself due to that, to ...that way of putting things. (Paula, Portuguese nurse) (Pereira 2007, 194).

The issues of precarious work and of being hired for short-term replacements are even more evident among Spanish nurses, particularly, among those from Catalonia. As is also true for Portuguese nurses, Spanish newly graduated nurses are the ones who mostly feel the changes in accessing work.

> Because when you start they don't give you a contract for a whole year, but give you a series of short contracts as a substitute. And so you probably go home one day, and you finish your contract and you say to yourself, 'I wonder

> when…?' And tomorrow morning they call you, 'please come' they say. The worst thing is the type of contracts. It's horrific at the beginning, because there are one-day contracts, two-day contracts, three-day contracts, or contracts where they only call you for the weekends, but they call you on Friday. Or they call you to come immediately. You can't have a life like that. On the other hand, what you want to do is work, but you don't have a life because you are always hanging about wondering whether they are going to call you or not. Of course if you say you can't and you say that you can't a lot of times, then they stop calling you. (Maite, Spanish nurse) (Müller et al. 2007, 207)

Older nurses with more stable contracts feel little or no impact of these measures. Having temporary replacement contracts is almost seen as normal during the early professional years. The medium time to get a permanent contract is around five years. Until then, it is more usual to find a short-term contract as well as to be rotated between institutions, according to institutional needs.

The professional implications of having short-term contracts frequently characterised by rotation between services and institutions are emphasised by nurses in some countries and place the quality of care at risk. Maite talks about her own experience:

> So today you are in neurology and tomorrow in gynaecology and the next day in general surgery… Of course you are the Jack of all trades and master of none: in other words, you know a little bit about everything, but you don't really know anything. You can't work with much security… (Müller et al. 2007, 207)

Such work situations do not facilitate professionals' integration in the working world. In her work, Benner (1984) transports Dreyfus' model of skills acquisition to the professional path of nurses. Her studies have allowed her to characterise five levels of nurses according to that model: novice, advanced beginner, competent, proficient and expert. The model defends the position that skill acquisition depends on contexts and experience and not on intelligence or personal gifts. Benner (ibid.) characterises as novice nurses not only new nurses but also those who are in the process of integrating in a new service (unit) and do not know the patients and the entire health context. In general, and as a form of protection, nurses at this level act according to the official rules and pre-established procedures. Such behaviour is limiting because strict rules may not always lead to a correct, expected and useful behaviour. Nurses at this level and at the following, advanced beginner, revise and re-orient their work since obtained experience may eventually lead to structuring practice in such a way that they become competent, when assessing the most and least important aspects of their work. Furthermore, Chang and Hancock (2003) also demonstrate that role ambiguity due to a lack of clear responsibilities is an important source of stress in the early months of work for new nurses. The fact that each ward has different personnel, management and routines can increase role ambiguity. Employers must re-examine their staffing levels so as to allow new-graduates to increase self-confidence and to provide for patients' physical and psychological needs (Chang & Hancock, 2003).

Nevertheless, some nurses mentioned as positive their exposure to different settings at the beginning of professional activity, since it widens the variety of situations with which professionals might have to deal and also it may work as a learning stimulus. However, taking into account patients' safety as the main goal and the stress it can cause to newly graduated nurses, it is questionable whether a wide work exposure is positive without the support of a truly positive environment. Such a positive environment is only possible when there are safety conditions, adequate staffing (in number and qualifications) and good learning conditions (Maurier & Northcott 2000; Stanton 2004; Stone et al. 2007; Lin & Liang 2007). However, most of the organizational restructuring in hospitals is carried out at a system level and is focused on managerial efficiency rather than on creating organizations that enable health care practitioners to deliver high quality care, which should be a priority (Aiken et al. 2002a).

Precarious conditions are not restricted to working conditions and to professional impact. This type of uncertainty, of lack of stability, also has consequences for personal life planning.

> It is. And I noticed that on a colleague of mine who entered one year ahead of me who was always under such a stress until she changed into an indefinite-term contract, my God, then there was the parents' stress, her stress, okay, people end up not having this stability to take that step forward and think about the future while they don't have professional stability. (...) for example, in that particular case I've just mentioned, at economical level, thinking of marrying.... having another life, buying a house, getting a car, because we face the risk of being sacked, there's always that thing, isn't that so? As things go nowadays... (Alexandra, Portuguese nurse) (Pereira 2007, 179).

As a consequence, when contracts are undefined, the impact of this uncertainty is responsible for direct worsening of young nurses' life conditions It seems that there is an unbalance between nurses' needs (and the special attention they require at the beginning of their professional life) and organizational demands, while competence and safety are two very important aspects not to be neglected.

Impact of Nurses' Working Conditions on Patients' Quality of Care

Work overload, stress from having to deal with concurrent needs, exhaustion, inability to care according to professional ideals are all factors that influence both the quality of the provided care and nurses' professional life. Due to the lack of staff, nurses need to set priorities in their actions, which brings out some conflicts between the professional role they consider appropriate and the part they actually play. This factor is quite relevant since nurses say that in the organization of their daily work, the dimension "own conception how work should be done" assumes a dominant part when considering which factors influence every day's nursing work (Solberg et al. 2007).

The decrease of required staff, whether it may be due to the attribution of new roles or because of new demands in terms of documentation and procedures, has an impact on nurses' professional and personal life, either because of lack of time or because of increasingly greater workload. All this leads to nurses gradually changing what they actually do in their professional settings. Whenever there is a need for reorientation of services in face of economic constraints, nurses' role may not be assured beyond providing physical care (Baumann 2007).

However, restructuring consequences can be also examined from patients' point of view. First, there are quality issues and the right to receive personal care as persons and not as clinical cases, according to the values they choose for themselves (Cody 2000). This right agrees with nursing theory. Second, the issue of patients' safety is very important. The relation between shortage of nurses, working conditions and risks for the patient has been well documented.

It is symptomatic that the International Council of Nurses (ICN) has set as motto for the Nurses International Day's celebrations themes such as: "Safe staffing saves lives" (2006); "Positive practice environments: quality workplaces = quality patient care" (2007) (Bauman 2007). Nurse shortage is global and it is one of the main factors that contribute to the deterioration of working environments. ICN reinforces the idea that safe staffing has positive impact on maintaining patients' quality care, on nurses' quality of life and on organizational results.

Oulton (2006) characterizes the following contributing factors to nursing shortage: Demand factors - ageing population, globalisation, public demands for service, and increasing mobility - and supply factors - unfavourable work environments such as workload, stress, burnout, little involvement in decision-making, and lack of support by management. Regarding the nurse/patients' safety balance, different studies found a positive connection between the increase in number of nurses and decrease of complications (urinary infections, pulmonary complications, sepsis, pressure ulcers, falls, strokes or reduction of deaths by specific reason) (Aiken et al. 2002b; Stanton 2004; ICN 2006).

Beyond staff issues, Rogers et al. (2004) have identified that both errors and near errors are most likely to occur in hospitals where nurses work twelve or more hours per shift. The use of extra hours and extended work shifts, due to nursing staff shortage, are also related to an increase of risk for patients. There was evidence of a significant increased risk in over 12 hours shifts, either due to extra work hours and to nurses working more than 40 hours per week (Rogers et al. 2004).

Furthermore high patient/nurse ratios (a normal procedure when health institutions try to cut costs) are associated with a greater risk of emotional exhaustion and dissatisfaction with work (Sheward et al. 2005)[7]. Such policies present risks for patients as well as for a poorer organizational climate. It was also evident that nurses, who work without adequate support, suffer poor health. Taking into account evidence that links nurse shortage with dissatisfaction with the workplace as having significant negative implications for patient safety, Lin and Liang (2007) defend

[7] However, unlike the data collected in our study, most nurses say they are pleased with the quality of care they are able to give.

the position that appropriate staff ratios are important but not sufficient. Nurses' satisfaction must be addressed and this can be achieved by empowering nurses by increasing their autonomy and status and by improving their working conditions. Stone et al. (2007) also found that nurses' working conditions are associated with patient safety outcomes. In a study developed in Intensive Care Units, they found that units with higher staffing presented lower infection rates, 30-day mortality and decubitus ulcer. They also found that increased overtime is associated with negative effects in all the above dimensions. These conclusions strongly suggest that the improvement of nurses' working conditions is an important issue for patients' safety. Thus, environments that are favourable to quality care depend on adequate staffing and nurses' appropriate qualifications and competence.

Nurses who suffer from stress, due to a heavy working schedule, problems with colleagues, inappropriate tasks or insecure working conditions, find it difficult to perform their tasks with high standards of quality care (Baumann 2006). The consequences of precarious work on professional practice are not much different from those previously stated when analysing nurse shortage, or, still, as it happened in the Greek case, with cyclical periods of shortage and integration of new professionals. On the one hand, there is a clear impossibility of giving quality holistic care, since nurse rotation gives neither the appropriate knowledge of patients nor it allows the nurturing of a long-term relationship.

> The worst thing is when you go from here to there you don't get to know any patient. The thing about the patients – they are very clever – and when they have never seen you then you are new. You are always new. So naturally, they don't trust you. Sometimes they trust more in what another person tells them that they have seen three days running than you, who are new, who they have just seen. (Maite, Spanish nurse) (Müller et al. 2007, 206)

On the other hand, the lack of boundaries makes impossible the development and the improvement of specific skills, something that may endanger patients' safety.

Thus, when talking about safe staffing, it may be necessary to look into the different characteristics beyond the number of nurses. One should consider concepts such as skill mix and assuring the balance between qualified and unqualified staff and of supervision (Needham, 1996 cited by Norrie & Goodson, 2007). For all these reasons, even though there are newly graduated nurses or immigrants available, they cannot fulfil nursing staff needs, since the safety of the care provided to patients might be at stake.

Though not directly related to the care provided, the generalised perception of a low salary contributes to a climate of low morale that may have an impact on quality of care. Salary issues are one of the global problems nursing faces in the new century, along with two other factors: status and morale (Pearson & Peels 2001). The voices of interviewed nurses help us better understand the reasons for dissatisfaction: an inappropriate salary for nurses' long training; the profession's physical and mental demands; and, mostly, the high level of responsibility required of them.

> You must know how to make independent decisions. We're dealing with people's health after all, so the decisions that we make are very responsible. (...) It's very hard physically, lifting patients and all. Taking all that into consideration, the responsibility and physical demands, the salary is too small. (Jenna, Finnish nurse) (Kosonen & Houtsonen 2007a, 276)

A Greek study conducted in 2000 also showed that in public hospitals the majority of nurses (32%) consider their low salaries as the most serious problem of working in public hospitals; 25% the shortage of nursing personnel; and only 9% the organization and functioning of hospitals[8].

One of the English nurses says that she earns as much as a mailman and Paula, from Portugal, chooses teaching as a term of comparison:

> My cousins earn more than I do, they work much less than me, they have much less responsibility than me, they surely don't get half as beat as I do and they earn a lot more than I do, but... it's unfair... but... that's it. I think we don't earn enough considering what we go through. (Paula, Portuguese nurse) (Pereira 2007, 174)

The mixture of high effort/low reward and the comparison with other professions makes the feeling of injustice more evident.

The Impact of Men's Entry into Nursing

The result of men's entry into the previously entirely feminine occupation of nursing has been another type of restructuring. Although restructuring is taking place in many of the studied countries[9], only three countries studies, UK, Ireland and Greece, document that men's entry in nursing has brought about a change in the name of nurses that has probably played more than just a symbolic role in improving the image of the profession. The change in the name was necessary because it was no longer possible to call nurses 'sisters', especially in Greece where the word "athelfes" (sisters) also refers to homosexual men[10]. This is a particularly sensitive issue since being stereotyped as "feminine" or outright as homosexuals plagues male nurses. At present the new term '*nosileftis*', [that we have translated as 'nurse' due to a lack of a better term in English], is used for both men and women with university training, while those with only a two-year training are called 'assistant *nosileftes*'. The importance of the name change lies in the fact that the Greek word '*nosileftis*' has a connotation of treatment (from the verb *nosilevo* that means to "treat"), of professional knowledge and of greater prestige.

---

[8] "Draft Law on the Creation of an Association of Greek Nurses and Other Provisions", Opinion of the Economic and Social Committee, Athens, Greece, 7 July 2004.

[9] For example, although in Portugal one in five nurses is male, the country study did not provide any relevant data.

[10] Now the previous term 'nosokomos' is only used to refer to hospital orderlies ('travmatioforis) who carry patients, wash them and perform other physical tasks.

Male and female Greek nurses consider that men's entry into the profession beneficial for the professionalization of nursing. They feel that men's entry in nursing is strategically important because it helps the profession to escape the marginal position usually accorded to "women's" occupations. Maria, the young Greek woman nurse said:

> I feel that the presence of men in the profession can help improve the image of the profession because men are more ambitious and more career-oriented. They try to continuously read, learn more things. There is a permanent male nurse in the ward and for a while there was also a contractual male nurse. Because in this ward there are only women patients, in the beginning some women patients were uncomfortable with a male nurse. Now I think that the situation has improved; the male nurse is accepted as well as the women nurses and some women patients even prefer the male nurse and some of them call him 'doctor' and show that they have more confidence in him than in the young women surgeons (Safiliou-Rothschild 2007, 162).

And Konstantinos, the male nurse, agrees:

> The presence of men in nursing has helped improve the professional image. Patients and their relatives confront differently men than women nurses and even relationships between men and women colleagues are different. It's different when only women work in nursing and different when there are also men. The changes are positive. When a profession is closed to the other gender, it's like a ghetto, not a good thing. Work conditions change when it opens up. Men may be able to perform some duties easier than women and vice versa. So the practical aspects of work change for the better (Safiliou-Rothschild 2007, 162).

Irish women nurses express similar positive views about the entry of men in nursing and feel that conditions improve when there is a better gender mix: "*in psychiatry it would be predominantly male you do find actually things improve, conditions improve, research will improve when there is a better gender mix...*"(Ellen, Irish nurse*)*.[11] In UK, a male nurse interviewed[12] reports that there is "female to male discrimination within nursing..." In more detail, he says:

> ...I mean, I think blokes get [the] stick...from some female nurses about, I mean a lot of it, there's all the kind of stereotypes, like...but the thing is, it can, it's openly expressed to me, I can't, you know, 'you can't multi-task' and people kind of quite regularly, it's sort of jokingly, it's jovial but it's like 'Oh, you know, you're useless at multi-tasking, you can't, or you're not very tidy, or you're not any good at cleaning'...But sometimes, I mean it gets a bit

[11] Primary data from Irish nurse's interview.

[12] Primary data from English male nurse's interview.

> frustrating. 'Oh, yeah, you know you are useless because you are male'...I do meet that, definitely, the kind of sexism, and I think almost it's different if you are gay. It's more, you're more, you are perceived as more effeminate, or you're more in touch with your feminine side and therefore maybe you can multi-task, therefore maybe all of the shortcoming of heterosexual males, you don't exist...

His comments seem to reflect reality since in UK the entry of male nurses constituting at least 10% of all nurses had led to a degree of relative marginalization of male nurses, who, at least in the early stages, constitute a minority, which was in some respects discriminated against. For example, there are research indications that male nurses, being a cultural and numerical minority within a female occupational group, are more stressed than women nurses, have higher rates of sickness absence than women nurses, report more work-related hassles than women nurses (Evans & Steptoe 2002) and are more exposed to violence than women nurses (Lawoko et al. 2004). Even in Norway, a country considerably advanced in gender equality, research shows that male nurses are more often exposed to bullying at work than their female colleagues, this finding persisting even after adjustment for a series of background factors (Eriksen & Einarsen 2004). In 2006, the existence of gender discrimination against male nurses was formally acknowledged in UK, when a former student male nurse won a landmark sex-discrimination case against NHS hospitals that did not permit him to perform intimate medical procedures on women patients, if a female chaperone was absent, while female nurses are permitted to provide intimate care to male patients with no chaperone required (Nursing Profession News 2006). Still in Ireland, it is reported that male nurses are often apprehensive about using physical touch and they use coping strategies in response to their fears of being accused of using touch inappropriately (Keogh & Gleeson 2006). Women patients in the gynaecological oncology ward with no prior experience of hospital admission or being cared by a male nurse, state that they prefer to be cared by a female nurse. However, the same does not hold true for women patients with previous hospital admission within the last five years or who have been cared for by a male nurse (Lodge et al. 1997). The transitory nature of women patients' aversion to male patients was also confirmed in the Greek study, since oncology women patients were reported to eventually prefer to be taken care by a male nurse (Safiliou-Rothschild 2007).

In the UK, male nurses experience challenges to their masculine identity from various sources and in a variety of ways. In response to these challenges, they develop strategies in order to accommodate their masculinity by either attempting to maintain a traditional masculinity by distancing themselves from female colleagues, and/or by partially (re)constructing a different masculinity by identifying with their non-traditional occupation. These responses work to maintain men as the dominant gender, even in these traditionally defined "women's jobs" (Cross & Bagihole 2002). Thus in UK, men are climbing the nursing career ladder much quicker than women, despite the fact that women have much longer experience in the profession and better nursing qualifications, according to research conducted by the Independent Policy

Studies Institute. This report, commissioned by the Department of Health shows that men were twice as likely to be serving in the higher nursing grades. This may be at least partly explained by the fact that just 5 percent of men and 45 percent of women work part-time (Policy Studies Institute 1998). Because women nurses continue to utilize part-time and flexible arrangements much more than men, they fall behind male colleagues in terms of career development and promotion prospects, with managers selecting males over females (particularly those who work part-time) regarding functional role allocation in the hospital setting. Thus, male nurses advance the development of their nursing careers more rapidly than women forming a disproportionate percentage of those in higher grades and management posts (Whittock et al. 2002). In addition, qualified female nurses feel more restricted than qualified men in their ability to take paid time off work, to go on training courses and to get course fees paid. Statistics in the UK show that while 93% of the nursing staff is women, men represent approximately 45% of all those who take up opportunities for higher education courses and accept senior/management positions (Royal College of Nursing 1995). Finally, women were more likely than men to work in specialties with limited chance for promotion, such as community nursing, while men are more likely to work in the area of mental illness or disability (Policy Studies Institute 1998). However, in the Greek university hospital studied, there was no male nurse in a supervisory position, probably because of the recent entry of men in significant numbers in the profession.

As the Greek male nurse predicts, it is quite possible that men's entry in nursing may further increase significantly:

> Still there are more women than men but the difference has decreased. In the following generations, it may change even more but I don't know whether it will ever happen to have more men than women. At least here in Greece, it's a good way for men to get a job faster than by studying other things. The prospective for jobs [in nursing] is good, so it's attractive for men (Konstantinos Greek nurse) (Safiliou-Rothschild 2007, 48).

It is expected that this process of "defeminization" will be completed when male nurses will constitute at least one-fourth of professional nurses with tertiary education and a considerable number of them will assume supervisory and management positions. Research in the U.S. has shown that men in women-dominated occupations benefit from the "glass elevator" phenomenon because men assist each other to rise up to high management positions (Williams 1992).

CONCLUDING REMARKS

Caring is often defined as providing physical, spiritual, emotional and social comfort to patients. It is considered to be at the *core* of nurses' professional identification and one of the main factors that appeal to nurses and lead them to choose the profession. It is also thought to be one of the main reasons for which they remain in the profession (Kosonen & Houtsonen 2007b).

As for professional identity, it is believed that nurses share one characteristic: they embrace a holistic philosophy of care and this philosophy shapes their work (Meleis 2007; Baumann 2007).

Increasingly, however, restructuring and particularly cost considerations change working conditions in nursing in such a way that nurses do not have the time and the possibility to care in a holistic way. Personnel shortage and precariousness of work oblige nurses to focus instead primarily on patients' immediate care. It seems reasonable to reach to the conclusion that nurses are not able to find the appropriate conditions to practice their work according to their professional ideals, because organizations do not share the view that these ideals are necessarily the core of nursing. In other words, nurses struggle to fulfil the social role they define as their own.

In fact, while holistic nursing care and patient advocacy remain important ideals for the nursing profession, institutional restructuring and changing working conditions often render difficult the realisation of these ideal professional standards. Nurses, therefore, who were educated and socialized to believe that holistic care was their primary role, may feel quite uncomfortable and frustrated. For many nurses, the transition away from the ideal of holistic care requires difficult changes in their conception of their primary role and in professional identification. This transition in professional identification may create more unease than changes in working conditions such as shortage of nursing personnel, nurse rotation, precariousness of contracts and increase of administrative procedures.

However, the development of technological knowledge in health care has had important consequences for the practice of nursing as well as for the practice of medicine. At present, ignoring improved health care techniques can result in inadequate or poor nursing care of patients. Increasingly, it seems that there is a need for balancing caring with curing (that is, caring with technological knowledge) in order for nurses to better perform their caring role.

Furthermore, in a wider context, one must pay attention to the significant entry of men in nursing which may be changing the caring equation. Men, who are not defined by nurturing stereotypes but rather by resourcefulness in finding solutions and by an ability to control situations, tend to appreciate more and to emphasize research, scientific and technical knowledge. This does not mean that they reject the caring aspect but they tend to conceive more this caring as mediated by scientific and technical knowledge. The transition, therefore, of the nursing profession away from a women's occupation most probably brings along a more balanced view of nurses' caring role that integrates scientific and technical health care knowledge as an equally important element of nursing care.

Nurses' dissatisfaction, on the other hand, with low salaries and low professional autonomy and status may diminish as these professional aspects improve with the transition of nursing away from a feminine occupation. Nursing is undergoing an important transition that does not seem to be welcome by all nurses because it requires readjustments and redefinitions. In all these transitions, patients' safety must be institutionally ensured, especially as more patients become aware of their rights and demand good care, according to their expectations.

REFERENCES

Aiken, L., Buchan, J., Sochalski, J., Nichols, B., & Powel, M. (2004). Trends in international nurse migration. *Health Affairs, 23*(3), 69-77.

Aiken, L., Clarke, S., & Sloane, D. (2002a). Hospital staffing, organization, and quality of care: cross-national findings. *Nursing Outlook, 50*(5), 187-194.

Aiken, L., Clarke, S., Sloane, D., Sochalski, J., & Silber, J. (2002b). Hospital nurse staffing and patient mortality, nurse burnout, and job dissatisfaction. *JAMA, 2888*(16), 1987-1993.

Baumann, A. (2007). *Positive practice environments: quality workplaces=quality patient care. Information and action tool kit.* Geneve: ICN.

Beach, D. (Ed.) (2005). *Welfare state restructuring in education and health care: Implications for the teaching and nursing professions and their professional knowledge.* Retrieved September 8, 2008, from http://www.profknow.net/files/results/Literature_Review_WP1_EU.pdf

Benner, P. (2001) *De iniciado a perito: excelência e poder na prática clínica de enfermagem.* Coimbra: Quarteto. (Portuguese translation from the 2001 English commemorative edition: *From novice to expert. Excellence and power in clinical nursing practice*, of 1984 Benner's work).

Chang, E., & Hancock, K. (2003). Role stress and role ambiguity in new nursing graduates in Australia. *Nursing and Health Sciences, 5*, 155-163.

Chen, K. (2000). The focus of the discipline of nursing: caring in the holistic human health experience. *Graduate Research in Nursing, 2*(1), 8.

Cody, W. (2000) Paradigm shift or paradigm drift? A meditation on commitment and transcendence. *Nursing Science Quarterly, 13*(3), 93-103.

Cross, S., & Bagilhole, B. (2002). Girls' jobs for the boys? Men, masculinity and non-traditional occupations. *Gender, Work and Organization, 9*(2), 204-226.

Dupont, M., & Sugrue, C. (2007). Irish nurses' work and life under restructuring: professional experiences, knowledge and expertise in changing contexts. In T. Kosonen & J. Houtsonen (Eds.) *European Nurses' Life and Work under Restructuring: Professional Experiences, Knowledge and Expertise in Changing Contexts* (pp. 90-146). Retrieved September 8, 2008, from http://www.profknow.net/files/results/D05_European_Nurses_Life_and_Work_under_Restructuring.pdf

Eriksen, W., & Einarsen, S. (2004). Gender minority as a factor of exposure to bullying at work: The case of male assistant nurses. *European Journal of Work and Organizational Psychology, 13*(4), 473-492.

Evans, O., & Steptoe, A. (2002). The contribution of gender-role orientation, work factors and home stressors to psychological well-being and sickness absence in male- and female-dominated occupational groups. *Social Science and Medicine, 54*(4), 481-492.

Goodson, I. & Norrie, C. (2005). *Welfare State Restructuring in Education and Health Care: Implications for the Teaching and Nursing Professions and their Professional Knowledge.* Retrieved September 8, 2008, from http://www.profknow.net/files/results/WP2.pdf

Houtsonen, J., Kosonen, T., Marrero, I., & Pereira, H. (2007, September). *European Nurses Life and Work under Restructuring.* Paper presented at ECER meeting, Ghent.

ICN - International Council of Nurses (2006). *Safe staffing saves lives. Information and action tool kit.* Geneve: ICN.

Keogh, G., & Gleeson, M. (2006). Caring for female patients: The experiences of male nurses. *British Journal of Nursing, 15*(21), 1172-1175.

Kosonen, T., & Houtsonen, J. (2007a). Finnish Nurses. In T. Kosonen & J. Houtsonen (Eds.) *European Nurses' Life and Work under Restructuring: Professional Experiences, Knowledge and Expertise in Changing Contexts* (pp. 259-279). Retrieved September 8, 2008, from http://www.profknow.net/files/results/D05_European_Nurses_Life_and_Work_under_Restructuring.pdf

Kosonen, T., & Houtsonen, J. (2007b). Nurses' Life and Work under Restructuring in seven European contexts – a comparative report. In T. Kosonen & J. Houtsonen (Eds.) *European Nurses' Life and Work under Restructuring: Professional Experiences, Knowledge and Expertise in Changing Contexts* (pp. 12-61). Retrieved September 8, 2008, from http://www.profknow.net/files/results/D05_European_Nurses_Life_and_Work_under_Restructuring.pdf

Kottow, M. (2001). Between caring and curing. *Nursing Philosophy, 2*(1), 53-61.

Lawoko, S., Soares, J., & Nolan, P. (2004). Violence toward psychiatric staff: a comparison of gender, job and environmental characteristics in England and Sweden. *Work and Stress*, *18*(1), 39-55.

Lin, L., & Liang, B. (2007). Addressing the nursing Environment to promote patient safety. *Nursing Forum*, *42*(1), 20-30.

Lodge, N., Mallett, J., Blake, P., & Fryatt, I. (1997). A study of gynaecological patients'perceived levels of embarrassment with physical and psychological care given by female and male nurses. *Journal of Advanced Nursing*, *25*(5), 893-907.

Maurier, W., & Nortcott, H. (2000). Job uncertainty and health status for nurses during restructuring of health care in Alberta. *Western Journal of Nursing Research*, *22*(5), 623-641.

Meleis, A. (2007). *Theoretical Nursing. Development and Progress* (4th ed.). Philadelphia: Lippincott Williams & Williams.

Müller, J., Larrain, V., Creus, A., Marrero, I., Muntadas, M., Hernandez, F., & Sancho, J. (2007). Case study report – Life Histories – Nurses Spain. In T. Kosonen & J. Houtsonen (Eds.) *European Nurses' Life and Work under Restructuring: Professional Experiences, Knowledge and Expertise in Changing Contexts* (pp. 199-226). Retrieved September 8, 2008, from http://www.profknow.net/files/results/D05_European_Nurses_Life_and_Work_under_Restructuring.pdf

Newman, M. (2002). The pattern that connects. *Advances in Nursing Science*, *24*(3), 1-7.

Norrie, C., & Goodson, I. (2007). English nurses' work and life under restructuring: professional experiences, knowledge and expertise in changing contexts. In T. Kosonen & J. Houtsonen (Eds.) *European Nurses' Life and Work under Restructuring: Professional Experiences, Knowledge and Expertise in Changing Contexts* (pp. 62-89). Retrieved September 8, 2008, from http://www.profknow.net/files/results/D05_European_Nurses_Life_and_Work_under_Restructuring.pdf

Nursing Profession News (2006, June 10). Justice to former male nurse in sex discrimination case. Retrieved September 10, 2008, from http://www.medindia.net/news/view_news_main.asp?x=11155

Oulton, J. (2006). The global nursing shortage: overview of issues and actions. *Policy, Politics & Nursing Practice*, *7*(3), 345-395.

Pearson, A., & Peels, S. (2001). Problems faced by Nurses. *International Journal of Nursing Practice*, 7(5), 521-525.

Pereira, H. (2007). Portuguese Nurses' lives under restructuring: case study report. In T. Kosonen & J. Houtsonen (Eds.) *European Nurses' Life and Work under Restructuring: Professional Experiences, Knowledge and Expertise in Changing Contexts* (pp. 169-198). Retrieved September 8, 2008, from http://www.profknow.net/files/results/D05_European_Nurses_Life_and_Work_under_Restructuring.pdf

Policy Studies Institute (1998). *Largest survey of nurses uncovers major gender inequalities*. Retrieved September 8, 2008, from http://www.psi.org.uk/news/pressrelease.asp?news_item_id=43

Rogers, A., Hwang, W., Scott, L., Aiken, L., & Dinges, D. (2004). The working hours of hospital staff nurses and patient safety. *Health Affairs*, *23*(4), 202-212.

Royal College of Nursing (1995). *Equality in Education*. London: Royal College of Nursing.

Safiliou-Rothschild, C. (2007). Greek nurses' work and life under restructuring: professional experiences, knowledge and expertise in changing contexts. In T. Kosonen & J. Houtsonen (Eds.) *European Nurses' Life and Work under Restructuring: Professional Experiences, Knowledge and Expertise in Changing Contexts* (pp. 147-164). Retrieved September 8, 2008, from http://www.profknow.net/files/results/D05_European_Nurses_Life_and_Work_under_Restructuring.pdf

Sheward, L., Hunt, J., Hagen, S., Macleod, M., & Ball, J. (2005). The relationship between UK hospital nurse staffing and emotional exhaustion and job dissatisfaction. *Journal of Nursing Management*, *13*, 51-60.

Sochalski, J. (2001). Quality of care, nurse staffing, and patient outcomes. *Policy, Politics & Nursing Practice*, *2*(1), 9-18.

Sohlberg, P., Czaplicka, M., Lindblad, S., Houtsonen, J., Müller, J., Morgan, M., Wärvick, G., Dupont, M., Norris, C., Kitching, K., & Kosonen, T. (2007). *Professional Expertise under Restructuring: Comparative studies of Education and Health Care (The survey study)*. Retrieved September 8, 2008, from http://www.profknow.net/files/results/WP3_Final_report.pdf

Stanton, M. (2004). Hospital nurse staffing and quality of care. *Research in Action*, *14*. Retrieved September 10, 2008, from http://www.ahrq.gov/research/nursestaffing/nursestaff.pdf

Stone, P., Mooney-Cane, C., Larson, E., Horan, T. Gance, L., Zwanziger, J., & Dick, A. (2007). Nurse Working conditions and patient safety outcomes. *Medical Care*, *45*(6), 571-578.

Wärvic, G. (2007). Nurses' life histories: the Swedish case. In T. Kosonen & J. Houtsonen (Eds.) *Nurses' Life and Work under Restructuring: Professional Experiences, Knowledge and Expertise in Changing Contexts* (pp. 227-258). Retrieved September 8, 2008, from http://www.profknow.net/files/results/D05_European_Nurses_Life_and_Work_under_Restructuring.pdf

Whittock, M., Edwards, C., McLaren, S. *et al*. (2002). "The tender trap": gender, part-time nursing and the effects of "family-friendly" policies on career advancement. *Sociology of Health and Illness*, *24*(3), 305-326.

Williams, C. (1992). The Glass Escalator: Hidden Advantage for Men in the "Female" Professions. *Social Problems*, *39*(3), 253-267.

GUN-BRITT WÄRVIK, RITA FOSS LINDBLAD
& MAEVE DUPONT

PATIENT ORIENTATION OF NURSES AND RESTRUCTURING OF HEALTH CARE

INTRODUCTION

> The medics give the instructions from a medical point of view and then they go themselves and the nurses instigate that or you arrange it or organize and you know you're talking to families you're talking to patients, you're counselling, you're everything you are, just basically are if you are not doing it yourself you are arranging for somebody else to do it so it's just a momentous role (Aideen).

The Irish nurse quoted above, Aideen, positions nurses at the centre of what often is referred to as a situations of patient oriented work, where she sees nurses as "momentous" mediators between patients, relatives, and other health care professionals. She refers to interactions with different people and things, and in the context of the aims of facilitating work with patients. Her workplace is a large university hospital where many other professional groups are employed, all with different kinds of training, jurisdiction, and organisational positions. Most likely, all these professionals would, like Aideen, point to patient orientation as a core of their work. However, Aideen indicates some of the complexities involved in nurses' work and the ways in which their relationships with patients are mediated and put to work.

The aim of this chapter is to explore some of the consequences of health care restructuring for Irish and Swedish nurses and their work, and by taking patient orientation of nurses as a point of departure. Indeed, patient orientation and "the patient at the centre" has been a primary goal of many ideas attached to health care restructuring in decades (Saltman 1992). Consequently, patient orientation of nurses brings up many questions about their competencies and professional identity, and the ways in which it relates to the routines and practices of nurses' work.

However, the everyday ease with which patient orientation can be understood is, from a conceptual as well as empirical point of view, far from simple. First, patient orientation can be regarded as a sociological concept of a relation, emphasising the close interaction between nurse and patient. This is about patient orientation as something that often goes together with normative theories of caring (Allen 2004), for instance, connected to ideas of holistic care (Levin 1971) or emotional labour (Erickson and Grove 2008). The focus is on nurses' work on a day-to-day basis.

J. Houtsonen, G.-B. Wärvik (Eds.), European Nurses' Life and Work Under Restructuring pp. 117-134.

Second, patient orientation of nurses can be discussed in terms of legislations and patient's rights (Vaartio & Leino-Kilpi 2005). For instance, health care professionals such as nurses are regulated in legislation; standards may be based on legislation, and demands on competences and formal education. Patients have the right to be given information and to be treated on equal terms by highly qualified professionals, as stated in the Swedish Health Care Act (HSL 1982: 763; see also An Bord Altranais 2000a, 2000b; The National Board of Health and Welfare 2005).[1] Here patient orientation means professional commitments to patient populations, but also to society as a whole. Third, patient orientation of nurses' work can also be seen from an economic point of view. The focus is then rather narrow, implying fairly radical and market-oriented transformations of health care services and the entire health care system. Patient orientation in this instance becomes a means of organisational change through the ("empowered") patient, who is converted into a customer whose demands should be met by (reconfigured) entrepreneurial professionals. A client-professional relationship based on trust then turns into a customer-entrepreneur relationship based on distrust, embedded in concerns for economic efficiency. The focus is on managerial needs of the health care organisation.

The main argument in this chapter is that these three aspects of patient orientation are important but should not be mixed up. We should avoid discussing one aspect of patient orientation, for instance, economisation of patients, by using another aspect, e.g. patients' rights in legislative terms and vice versa. One reason is ethical, that the three aspects mentioned above are often treated in an indistinct way in the public health care debate, a topic that will be discussed further in the next section. Another reason is for analytical comparative purposes, to better understand the consequences of health care restructuring from the perspective of nurses.

PATIENT ORIENTATION AND HEALTH CARE RESTRUCTURING

Recent decades have been described as a period of health care restructuring with implication for nurses' work. Ireland and Sweden are no exceptions (Beach 2005; Kosonen and Houtsonen 2007). An overall state and management-driven ambition is to raise the efficiency of services. Techniques of different kinds have been introduced with the idea of creating restructuring dynamics in the everyday practice of health care and in terms of de-regulation, privatisation, marketisation, auditing, etc. (e.g. Dent 2003; Sen 2003). These broad changes in financing, governing and production of health care are also connected to ideas of patient orientation, meaning a market-driven strengthening of patient power.

[1] The Irish An Bord Altranais (ABA) is a statutory body that provides for the registration, control and education of nurses and is responsible for the regulation of nursing practice. The National Board of Health and Welfare (Socialstyrelsen) is the Swedish supervisory body for health care, including regulation, monitoring and evaluation. The tasks of the Board also cover registration of health care professionals, including nurses.

In particular, Richard B. Saltman, an American professor of Health Policy and Management, has been an influential debater concerning strategies for the development of European health care systems. In the following, we will therefore briefly explore some of his ideas. On his agenda has been the aim of influencing policymakers and thereby forcing change. For instance, Saltman and his co-writers argue that the following overarching objectives have "played a role in most recent European national election campaigns" (Figueras et al. 2002, xi):

- Universal access for all citizens
- Effective care for better health outcomes
- Efficient use of resources
- High-quality services
- Responsiveness to patient concerns

The list includes universal rights for the citizens. It is a good list; of course, we all want high quality health care with universal access. We want to get effective treatments when we are ill and most of us also want to meet health care professionals who listen to our point of view. No one in the Western world would expect health care services supplied randomly. These rights are also protected by legislation and, for instance, by state regulation of nurses' work and demands on formal competencies.

However, the main concern of the list is better health care for less money, i.e. economic incentives to change practice and the professional configuration and one solution is presented as the one and only way, namely the patient. The patient in this instance does not refer to a relation, the close interaction between professional and client; it is the patient as the economic resource. Saltman (1992) identifies several pressures for reform, which are often repeated in the everyday health care debate: an ageing population, a changing panorama of diseases with an increasing number of chronically ill and disabled, new advanced treatments and technologies and rising expectations of the public when it comes to services. His answer, also adopted in the everyday debate, is to let the money follow the patient. Saltman argues against what he sees as a rigid and inflexible health care bureaucracy and says that the only way forward is to hand over power to the patient. Responsiveness to the citizens/users is emphasised (cf. Du Gay and Salaman 1992). Patients are not depicted as passive recipients of care, but as autonomous and well-informed users of health services, involved in decision making (Coulter and Magee 2003). This is, however, not the same as universal commitment to a patient population and health care on equal terms, where services are distributed by professionals according to individual needs. The health care professionals are distrusted. The caring nurse is accepted but only if acting like an entrepreneur. The nurse specialists are cheaper than doctors and sometimes put forward as substitutes for doctors. Similarly, assistant nurses are cheaper than nurses. As for instance, discussed by Eva Bejerot (2008) in a Swedish context, the idea of "the patient at the centre" includes far-reaching state/managerial ambitions to change the relations between clients, health care staff and management.

Taken together, we get a restructuring situation with a focus on clients *and* results. This is, of course, something very different to patient orientation as a focus on the unique individual needs of the client or patient orientation as an aspect of solidarity and universal rights. To use the title of a report edited by Saltman et al. (2002), "Regulating entrepreneurial behaviour in European health care systems", patient orientation refers here to a new role of the state (Saltman 2002). Relations between state and professionals are meant to be re-regulated by means of re-configured incentives.

> The State pursues these objectives through a complex and finely nuanced mix of mandatory requirements – sticks – and behavioural inducements – carrots. This mix of requirements and inducements can be direct or indirect, and may also be intentional or unintentional in nature (Saltman 2002, 1677-1678).

Studies of such re-regulated relations between the state, professionals and citizens, and the meaning given to these changes by front-line professional actors, have been a point of departure in the PROFKNOW project and, hence, an essential question in this chapter is how regulating measures operate on the patient orientation of nurses, taking into account its relational, legislative and economic aspects.

CONSTITUTING "THE PATIENT" – AN ANALYTICAL TOOL WHEN STUDYING PATIENT ORIENTATION OF NURSES AND RESTRUCTURING

Patient orientation as a focus on relations and the individual needs of the patients is a recurrent theme in the PROFKNOW life history reports, and is a highly valued aspect of nurses' professional identity. However, at the same time, the PROFKNOW studies also conclude that the nurses are not able to give the kind of care they want to. They do not have time to be with the patients as much as they should, or they are not able to carry out the kind of nursing care that they say they should be able to, according to their professional values. The focus is on the needs of the individual patient. Intensification of workload, haste and lack of resources are characteristic aspects of their daily work and sources of dissatisfaction (Kosonen and Houtsonen 2007). It is also quite easy to connect these tensions expressed by nurses to single restructuring aspects, such as shortage of nurses, economic regulating incentives and cutbacks, and to changes in nurse education, etc.

In the PROFKNOW project, we have analysed texts on restructuring as system narratives, i.e. discourses about ongoing changes in the context of health care institutions. In a similar way, we have analysed nurses' stories about their work and life as "working life narratives". The system narratives of restructuring and change are, according to their design strategy, supposed to have an impact on the work of nurses. However, we have tried to capture working life and restructuring, not as implementation of ideas with certain possible effects on institutions, but by paying close attention to the nurses' point of view, to the meanings nurses give to working life changes. Consequently, restructuring tools and strategies and how they are translated in the working life of nurses (Goodson & Lindblad 2008) are important in our analysis.

The idea here is not to construct nurses as victims of external restructuring forces. For instance, as mentioned above, we know from the life history reports (Kosonen and Houtsonen 2007) that the nurses talk about their situation as strained. This is, of course, a true situation; most likely, we can believe the nurses when they say that there is a lack of resources and when they describe their situation as frustrating. However, if we focus on restructuring as singularities, and on restructuring as objectified phenomena with clear and well-defined meanings, we might miss the kind of situations underlying the nurses' frustration.

Paying attention to the patient as differently constituted in the interaction with nurses is one possible way of studying the implications of health care restructuring for nurses' work, and of acquiring a better understanding of all the aspects of circumstances of patient orientation. In health care, the patient often tends to be a rather taken-for-granted category. In research and policy formulations of different kinds, the patient is stable and rarely questioned. However, we would argue that within the healthcare system generally, the patient shifts in terms of meaning as well as references. For example, patients can refer to "a sick lady in a hospital bed with critical difficulties in breathing", "people in a waiting room asking for planned services" as well as to "the printed result of a blood test from the laboratory" or "people to be mindfully scheduled for X-ray". The point of departure taken here is that the patient as a category is constituted, acquires its meaning and references, in practice, and the category is therefore highly dynamic, shifting from moment to moment when, for instance, encountering nurses, as in our cases.

In health care, as in other institutions, we can find fairly standardised procedures. These are all involved in the constitution of the patient and thereby also in the constitution of professional identities and competencies of the nurses. To mention just a few examples, there are action plans and outlines of different kinds about procedures when a patient is admitted to a hospital ward; preparation of patients for an X-ray examination; monitoring of patients after surgery and what can be expected and what should not be expected, etc. Commonly, nurses are the ones responsible for organising work so that all these processes run smoothly (Blomgren 2003). For instance, in her review of field studies of nurses' work, Davina Allen (2004) points to nurses as intermediaries of the health care organisation and argues that:

> The predominant focus of nursing work is not on individuals, but on patient populations and this general observation seems to hold true across a range of health care contexts (Allen 2004, 274).

Standards are efficient ways of processing people to manage the flow of patients through the health care system (Allen 2004) but also when handling the unique needs of the single patient.

As discussed earlier in this chapter, restructuring measures are often developed with the intention that they should influence a certain kind of patient orientation of health care professionals, meaning configuration of a more entrepreneurial outlook. Consequently, by acknowledging the complexities of nurses' patient orientation, we will in the following discuss some everyday and very ordinary examples of nurses' work, and ask: How is the patient orientation of nurses constituted when encountering patients? Are economic incentives linked to the patient orientation of nurses, and if so, how?

Our analysis concerns two kinds of situations. The first situation refers to nurses paying attention to individual needs of individual patients. The focus here is in particular on the nursing process and documentation. The second situation refers to nurses' management of the flow of the patient population. Here, the main focus is on aspects of teamwork as a restructuring tool. Finally we also discuss economy and patient orientation.

In this chapter, we have studied two different European health care contexts, Ireland and Sweden, but also two quite different kinds of health care settings. The Irish case study (Dupont & Sugrue 2007) concerns nurses and their work in a large university hospital. The hospital has a bed complement of over 600 beds and a staff of more than 2,000.[2] The Swedish case study (Wärvik 2007) concerns nurses and their work in a primary care centre in a multicultural context and a staff of around 60.[3]

The two case studies are based on life history interviews with nurses. Three nurses have been interviewed twice in each country and also been shadowed by the researchers during a total of nine full working days in each country. The Swedish case study also includes a group interview with four other nurses at the same workplace. The Irish nurses interviewed are Aideen, who is a nurse manager, Ellen, who is a clinical nurse specialist, and Nora, who is a staff nurse. The Swedish nurses are Anna and Nancy, both primary care nurses, and Nina, who is a district nurse. All three Swedish nurses are specialist nurses in different areas.

THE INDIVIDUAL NEEDS OF THE PATIENT

We will introduce this section by describing some fairly mundane events from nurses' work on monitoring individual patients and where nurses make use of their senses but also clinical chemical tests, etc. when constituting the patient. We will also introduce the two different contexts of nurses' work, the Irish hospital and the Swedish primary care centre.

---

[2] The Irish hospital is the principal undergraduate and post-medical training and research institute. There are two main sources of admission to the hospital, emergency cases transferred by ambulance or elective patients referred by general practitioners or other hospital doctors for specialised treatment.

[3] Swedish primary care was developed in the 1970s and 1980s as a way of breaking the dominance of the large-scale hospitals. Primary care centres are outpatient clinics and are intended mainly for emergency visits and long-term follow-up of patients. These centres have different categories employed: district nurses, primary care nurses, doctors, assistant nurses, physiotherapists, social workers, occupational therapists, psychologists, etc.

The Irish Hospital Ward and the Swedish Primary Care Centre

During interviews, the Irish nurse Aideen mentions the need for nurses to be very observant of their patients because nurses are the patients' advocates. She also says that this is particularly relevant after a patient has had surgery:

> A lot of our patients they would have after their surgeries they would often have problems talking...they would be dysphasic...so they might know what they want to say but they can't get the words out right or can only get some of the words out right so like you would have to be very observant, clued in, sensitive like pick up on non verbal cues (Aideen).

In her account, the biomedical condition of the patient is blurred with the physical manifestation of the postoperative state and the patients' life-situation. When the patient has problems communicating verbally, the nurse says that it is her job to be observant and try to understand.

Another example (from shadowing) of nurses' monitoring is the Irish nurse Nora who noted that a patient's arm was swollen because the intravenous drip-feed (IV line) was going into his tissue rather than his vein. The patient's failure to complain about the pain in his arm indicated that he was unable to verbally communicate his discomfort and therefore needed to be closely monitored. Nora's monitoring of the patient indicated bodily manifestations of his biomedical condition but also of a medical-technical intervention, namely the IV line. Here, she is doing something the patient under normal conditions would have been able to do without help, that is, complain about pain in his arm. His swollen arm was noticed at the same time as Nora, for some reason, observed another change in the patient's wellbeing, namely drowsiness.

The situations described above are rather banal episodes in the nurses' daily work. They are situations involving nurse/patient bedside interaction where the focus is on the unique needs of the individual patient. The patient emerges as conditions to be monitored by nurses, who pay attention to both the expected and the unexpected, not only to biomedical matters. These situations are held together by nurses. The patient is subjected to close monitoring due to a fairly short-term impairment of vital functions in a postoperative situation in life, a rather common hospital ward situation.

However, the patient orientation of nurses with a focus on the individual needs of individuals does not only concern short-term episodes of monitoring patients. The Swedish district nurse Nina says that an important aspect of her work at the primary care centre is helping patients to take charge of their chronic illness. For instance, her work includes long-term follow-up of patients with diabetes. During interviews, Nina talks about patients as being responsible for their own care. She thus depicts a kind of situation that differs from the postoperative monitoring situation on the surgical ward at the emergency hospital.

The following are notes from fieldwork and Nina's outpatient consultancy. She sees a patient with diabetes. Even this example is chosen to represent a normal episode in her patient oriented work:

Patient:[4] My test-results are not so good.

Nina: Okay.

Patient: /…/ I think about it all the time, the food. But it's hard. My blood sugar has been around eleven in the mornings. I don't know why it's so high in the mornings.

Nina: Do you eat in the evenings?

Patient: I try not to eat after eight o'clock, but it's difficult. I'm so hungry in the evenings.

Nina explains a connection between eating in the evenings and high morning blood sugar.

Patient: I would need appointments with you all the time, then I would shape up.

/…/

Nina analyses blood and urine in the lab to check glucose. She tells me that the test-results are too high.

/…/

Nina: Have you brought your diary?

Patient: No, I haven't used the diary that much.

Like the situations in the Irish hospital, this is about monitoring patients, but in a Swedish primary care setting, an outpatient clinic. The focus is on the patient with a disease, with all its potential implications. Specifically, the focus is on the patient's biochemical condition (blood sugar) in this selection from the field notes and both the nurse and the patient play an active role, monitoring the diabetes. When monitoring, both Nina and the patient have access to clinical chemical tests as well as the patient's own statements about health-related issues. Nina could also have had access to the patient as a biochemical condition over a lengthy period if the patient had "used the diary". The diary contains blood and urine tests but also eating, exercise and other aspects of daily living of concern when checking the progress of a disease. The tests, the diary (monitoring at a distance) and the patient's expressions of (mis)behaviour are among Nina's tools when constituting the unique patient with specific needs. As in the Irish case above, these are also tools constituting interaction with a client.

In the next section, we discuss documentation as a tool for constituting the patient. The patient-orientation of nurses then also takes place within a legislative framework, although still emphasising the unique needs of the individual patients.

[4] The patient has given the researcher permission to participate.

Documentation Tools

During an interview, the Swedish nurse Nancy answers a question about the transformation of her work as a nurse. She describes a past not that glorious for nurses with a focus on work tasks and not on patients. "We didn't have a plan, we had no goals for our measures, things were just done and that was it", she says. Her work has changed for the better, Nancy argues, and concludes by saying that nurses today do their work with the patients' needs as the point of departure. Nurses then set goals for their nursing interventions and these goals are evaluated and can be changed over time. We can find similar reasoning in research on nurses' work. For instance, David Armstrong (1998) argues, when analysing the nurse-patient relationship as presented in influential nursing literature from the 1960s and 1970s, that the interaction between the two parties was decried as mechanistic and the patients presented as biological objects. Nancy refers to what is sometimes termed "the nursing process" (see e.g. de la Cuesta 1983), a phenomenon often used to describe a shift in nurses' patient orientation, from what often is termed task-orientation to a patient-centred approach (Smith 1998). The discursive shift in nurses' work also creates a dichotomy: now and then, the patient's need and body, the relation with the patient and the work task, the good nurse and the bad one.

However, we have to be cautious and not directly draw the conclusion that this dichotomy is only about the creation of professional relations versus ignorance and lack of empathy. Indeed, nursing has always been about caring but different periods have had their particular focus and vocabulary when describing nurses' work (Armstrong 1998). Instead, we may argue that the dichotomisation creates a situation where the very idea of a patient is changing, from a person who, for instance, should be prepared for surgery, or should have antibiotics in his vein, to a person with certain needs to assess, plan, deliver (care regarded as adequate by the nurse) and evaluate. These ideas also go together with tools for documentation of work.

Like the Swedish nurses, the Irish nurses talk about their work in terms of assessment, planning, delivery and evaluation of care of patients. The Irish nurse Nora describes the basic nursing skills as being the most essential. According to her, these skills are associated with a model of nursing (Activities of Living) developed by Roper, Logan and Tierney (1985). 'Activities of Living' describes the functional status of a person. According to the model, there are twelve activities of living, namely: Maintaining a Safe Environment, Communication, Breathing, Eating and Drinking, Elimination, Washing and Dressing, Thermoregulation, Mobilization, Work and Play, Expressing Sexuality, Sleeping, Death and Dying. Thus, the nursing process here involves assessing the patient's activities of living needs, planning how to attend to each need, delivering appropriate care and subsequently evaluating such care. For example, Nora is observed assessing a patient as having mobilization needs following a surgical procedure. She then plans how to prevent the complications from lying in bed (such as the development of deep vein thrombosis) and delivers the appropriate care. In this instance, she walks the patient up and down the ward and gives him so-called TED socks to wear to improve his circulation. Nora evaluates the patient's progress at regular intervals. She describes these aspects as the most essential nursing skills and thereby also depicts the need of the patient as being at the centre of her work.

The ideas behind the nursing process, often regarded as imported from the United States, were developed during the 1970s (de la Cuesta 1983) and introduced in many European countries on a broad basis during the 1980s. The process itself is, of course, not exceptional, or even unique to nursing. Presented as consisting of phases, it is clear that this is a common way of describing work flows in many other areas. However, over the decades there has also been an increasing emphasis on documentation of nurses' work. Nurses are required to keep patient records within a legal and ethical framework, both in Ireland and in Sweden. These records often follow the steps of the nursing process. Therefore Nora, in the example of the patient with mobilisation needs, records the results of a patient's assessment. She also documents how she plans to deliver care and systematically evaluates such care and the particular patient's progress. These care plans were first introduced in this Irish hospital in the early 1990s.

Documentation of patient oriented activities is also an aspect of the Swedish nurses' work at a primary centre. The Swedish nurse Anna says that nurses' documentation per see is nothing new, referring to her previous hospital work:

> Yes we documented earlier too, we wrote a lot in the intensive care unit, everything we did with the patients, reports to the nurse on night duty, what had happened to the patients. But it was rather arbitrary with our own words and so on.

Anna argues that documentation today is more precise, that there is a standard to be followed:

> Anna: The documentation became more precise, what do you refer to when you use that word? So it could be used internationally in a report, so we all know what we referred to when we used a word that everybody referred to the same thing. /.../.
>
> Interviewer: Internationally, you mean
>
> Anna: Yes in the different models that were growing. The VIPS model, you got search terms and so on.

Anna refers here to the so called VIPS model (an acronym for the Swedish words for Well-being, Integrity, Prevention, Safety), an analytical documentation model developed by Swedish nurse researchers as a field of research and published in 1991 (Ehnfors et al. 1991) "with the aim of supporting the systematic documentation of nursing care and promoting individualized care" (Ehrenberg et al. 1996, 853). The model is nowadays widely used in Swedish health care (Björvell et al. 2002), and is based on ideas about the nursing process. Ehrenberg et al. argue that the concepts used in the model "were a compromise between clinically oriented everyday nursing language and internationally recognized, professional terms" (Ibid., 854) and states further that "the endeavour in the development work was to focus on the content with relevance for patient care rather than the structure and format of records". The researchers also argue that "another focus was on patients' functioning in the activities of daily life rather than pathophysiological problems" (Ibid., 854).

We will not present the model in full here. The point to be made, however, is that the VIPS model, like the model developed by Roper, Logan and Tierney, offers a standardised language with reference to nurses' work. In this way, a patient is constituted as something towards which nurses' work can be oriented within a legislative framework of mandatory documentation. The models are, however, developed by nurses not only to describe nurses' competencies but also to change them (Ehnfors et al. 1998). Consequently, these models offer opportunities for development of what should be seen as nurses' work. The planning of the work process and the documentation models place the nurse very close to the patient, an analytical/monitoring caring position, also talked about as highly valued when nurses are interviewed in this study.

MANAGING THE FLOW OF THE PATIENT POPULATION

When discussing health care restructuring, it is important to remember that hospital care is no longer a place for convalescents. For instance, it is generally accepted today that medical and technological advances lasting recent decades are the reason why many badly injured persons and patients suffering from serious diseases survive today. Survival also often requires more advanced hospital care. However, the advances also mean that many patients earlier treated in hospitals nowadays are treated as (less expensive) out-patients in clinical settings or primary care. The hospitals wards are highly specialised, and so are the Irish nurses being interviewed here. At the same time, the number of hospital beds has been rapidly decreasing. Patients admitted to hospitals can therefore be expected to be also more demanding as regards nursing care.

Beside the medical and technological advances, there are also economic interests included in the changes in the panorama of diseases. For instance, a typical hospital patient stays for a shorter period today due to demands on effectiveness. Diagnostic procedures and treatments are required by management to be carefully planned in terms of efficiency of patient preparation, thus avoiding an extra patient day in hospital. Teamwork and cross-professional cooperation are often discussed as a means of promoting efficiency, particularly in the case of primary care (Saltman et al. 2006). The debate here concerns above all the work of General Practitioners but also involves nurses, for instance nurse specialists (Boerma 2006).

An argument in this section is that nurses with their middle position in the healthcare hierarchy are also positioned as mediators, organisers of efficiency concerning the flow of the patient population, and that this aspect is integrated in their workflow when interacting with patients (see also Allen 2004; Blomgren 2003).

Team Work – Patients of Nursing Care and Patients of Others

A patient care episode, be it in a hospital or in primary care, or both, often involves different health care actors whose actions have to be coordinated. For instance, a patient admitted to hospital, or who visits a primary care centre, meets nurses, but also doctors and assistant nurses. The patient also often meets other staff categories such as physiotherapists, occupational therapists, psychologists, social workers, laboratory staff, etc. This means that the flow of patients also has to be coordinated with the schedules of the actual patient population in mind.

By taking nurses' work as a point of departure we might argue that the workflows of the other staff categories intersect when the needs of the patient extend outside nursing care. The documentation models of nurses (see previous section) become standardising devices in use, indicating what should be regarded as nursing care and what should be handed over to doctors. The focus is on nurses' monitoring and assessment of the individual patient's needs as well as the individual planning of care. Teamwork in this instance means that the patient is constituted by legislation and/or institutionalised conventions connected to each staff group and that the nurses are organisers and coordinators of the efforts.

The Irish nurse Aideen talks about nurses organising such relations.

> And get the speech therapist involved and make sure that those kinds of referrals go in and that people…all the different allied health care professionals that can help the patient are involved (Aideen).

The Irish clinical nurse specialist Ellen talks about her activities in terms of "indirect care". She tries to influence others in their provision of "direct care". For example, following her assessment of patient's needs she plans the actions that are required and, if within her scope of practise, delivers the appropriate care. Frequently, Ellen's assessment leads to the provision of direct care, delivered by others. For instance, she might recommend a patient to visit his/her general practitioner for a blood test to check levels of medication. However, while Ellen might influence others in their provision of direct care she is constrained by a number of institutional conventions. For example, the psychology and psychiatry departments do not accept referrals from nurses. Therefore she has to go through a doctor to get one.

Similarly, the Swedish primary care nurse Anna talks about her work as the first patient contact at the primary care centre, work that also includes making triage decisions:

> And our task is to give them (the patients) an appointment time or not give them an appointment time, give advice, sometimes to tell them to come back for a follow-up, we can book visits to the district nurses, and in cases of emergency to the psychologist or social worker, for example, if the patient expresses suicidal tendencies. We usually send these patients to an emergency psychiatric clinic but sometimes you don't dare do that, because you have a feeling that the patient has serious suicidal thoughts (Anna).

Anna says that she organises the contacts the patient might need. She even makes an assessment of the patients' psychological condition and cannot just tell the patient to visit a psychiatric emergency clinic if, for example, she suspects that the patient has suicidal tendencies. When using the example about patients with suicidal tendencies to explain her job to the interviewer, she also positions herself as a mediator of health care, so the patient will come into contact with the right category of staff.

Besides being the first contact and making triage decisions, the Swedish primary care nurses also see patients with chronic illness on a consultancy basis for long-term follow-ups including diagnostic procedures. During fieldwork, Nancy refers to legislation and says she is not allowed to prescribe medication. When she notices that a patient would benefit from changes in medication, she contacts the doctor on behalf of the patient to get a prescription, or she books a visit to the doctor for the patient. However, organising collaboration between nurses and doctors is not always unproblematic according to Nancy. She talks about doctors and nurses as having separated work flows. There are no smooth routines available. In the following quote, the nurse Nancy talks about herself as being responsible for arranging a meeting with the doctor but also that the doctor is often occupied with her own business, i.e. seeing (other) patients.

> You can't get hold of them and sit down and talk to them, they never have time. And grabbing them in the corridor, I just don't want to do that. Because then their minds are somewhere else. We communicate with the help of the computer (Nancy).

The nurse is positioned close to the patient to do the monitoring and follow-up work. She takes it on herself to solve the situation, to be the mediator between patient and doctor. The patient, as constituted by and through nurse interventions, has to be transformed into a patient of the doctor so that he can get another type of care than that provided by the nurse. This is done with, among other things, the help of the schedule in the computer.

The idea of a primary care patient changes, from "the patient of nursing care" to "the patient of doctor's care", a transformative teamwork situation that appears fairly frequently at the primary care centre studied as a result of legislation concerning professional work tasks and institutional conventions, and often with nurses as mediators of efficiency.

Until now, we have discussed nurses' work and patient orientation on a day-to-day basis by taking the needs of the individual and the management of the flow of the patient population as points of departure. Our analysis has concerned relational and legislative aspects of patient orientation. In the next section, we will discuss implications of economisation of relations with patients, and how economic incentives are attached to the patient orientation of nurses.

ECONOMY AND PATIENT ORIENTATION

As discussed above, documentation is a powerful tool when constituting the individual needs of a patient but also when managing the flow of patients. The digital patient record, the VIPS model, used by the Swedish nurses is part of a computer system for organising work with patients and communication between staff. In addition, this system is linked to the economy system, meaning that working with patients also involves making economic calculations. Everything registered in the patient record also generates economic information. This means that the patient orientation of nurses always has economic implications. The patients add resources to the workplace in line with purchasing procedures.

These purchasing procedures regulate the number of patients this Swedish primary care centre should see. The patient becomes the axis of resources at the same time as these resources are limited as regards the time available for each patient. As mentioned, restructuring incentives are built into the digitalised patient record system and thus are also attached to the work process of nurses (and doctors). From the perspective of the nurses, we get a situation of time management where the needs of the individual patient are in conflict with the citizens' need of easily available health care. Thus, a tension in nurses' work is also created when, for instance, as in the Swedish life history report, the nurses were confronted with a patient with rather serious health-related problems and a limited number of appointment times to see a general practitioner at the same time as they were obliged by management not to refuse anyone in need of care. The situation was very frustrating for the nurses. According to the nurses, many patients needed a longer period to see a doctor than the specified fifteen minutes but if they gave the patients, for instance, 30 minutes there was less time available for appointments for the patient population (Wärvik 2007).

The economic incentive in the Irish hospital setting works in a somewhat different way. For instance, the nurse manager Aideen talks about management-oriented aspects of her work and demands on efficiency. At the same time, the Irish nurses talk about a shortage of nurses and a limit to the recruitment of full-time staff and limited resources that have impacted on each nurse, as discussed in the Irish life history report (Dupont and Sugrue 2007). Their workload is both heavy and demanding as a consequence of the lack of manpower, they argue. Auxiliary nurses have been employed on the hospital wards, meaning that they take over parts of the nurses' work on patients' basic nursing care.[5] In addition, a large number of international nurses have been recruited in order to cope with the shortage of nurses. It appears, however, that their introduction has not been without problems. For instance, they only get six weeks to acclimatise to the Irish system. This is possibly inadequate, given that they come from different cultures and training systems.

---

[5] In Swedish hospitals, this process took place during the 1960s with auxiliary nurses and assistant nurses replacing nurses for efficiency reasons. Since around the mid-1980s, the Swedish situation has been the reverse, assistant nurses positions are converted into nurse positions (Lannerheim 1995).

However, the resources are not directly attached to the individual patient. Economic resources in this instance refer to manpower planning and thus, Aideen moves people between hospital wards to cope with fluctuating workloads and case complexity. The resources are not attached to the individual patient per se, such as adding resources to the ward, but here the patient population of the ward is a point of departure. The budget and the staffing plan are in the hands of Aideen and she also faces pressure from hospital management to reduce, for instance, the number of agency staff when spending has reached a certain limit. Aideen keeps expenditure within budget by means of a monthly review. From the perspective of nurses, we get a situation where the pressure from the needs of the individual patient is built into the work process but not the citizens' need of health care. The state operates here more indirectly by setting the budget for the hospital's nursing care.

CONCLUDING COMMENTS

In this chapter, we have addressed some of the consequences for nurses of health care restructuring. We have drawn on two life history reports of the PROFKNOW project and thus also two different nurse settings: an Irish university hospital and a Swedish primary care centre. By focusing on everyday situations in nurses' work, we have taken the relational, legislative and economic aspects of patient orientation of nurses into account. For analytical purposes, we have also concentrated on two main characteristics of the everyday work of nurses: the needs of the individual patient and the management of the flow of patients.

By separating these aspects of patient orientation and nurses' work, we can make a cross-table (table 1) to be used for comparative purposes. We want to make it clear that the comparisons do not, of course, refer to the two health care systems but to situations described in our two case studies, and only on a conceptual level. The cross-table helps us to identify tensions related to the restructuring of health care.

Table 1. Patient orientation of nurses and restructuring.

Aspect of nurses' work	Patient orientation		
	Relation	Legislation	Economy
The individual need of the patient	Irish case study: New division of labour with unclear boundaries and areas of competencies between nurses and nurse assistants (and foreign nurses).		Irish case study: Manpower planning.
Managing the flow of the patient population		Both cases: What is seen by nurses as universal and legislative rights of patients does not correspond with the lack of resources (lack of manpower and appointment times, respectively).	Swedish case study: Patients as economic resource.

To conclude, in the Irish case study, and on the hospital ward, we found tensions regarding the individual needs of the patient and patient orientation as the relation. Economic incentives affect the Irish nurses in a more indirect way and are connected to manpower planning. When the nurses talk about their work, they describe a shift from overall care to delivery of more specific "nursing care". There is a division of labour between nurses and auxiliary nurses. However, the analysis indicates that the boundaries between them are not fixed and that there are several grey zones where the work of the two might intersect. Due to the shortage of nurses, foreign nurses, with their education and experiences from another health care system, have been employed. This also causes tensions and blurred boundaries as regards identities and competencies (see table 1).

As regards managing the flow of patients, we found tensions in both case studies relating above all to legislation and the rights of the patients. Nurses are in an organisational intermediary position, and they are occupied with distribution of resources to the population of patients, a position that is thus sensitive to lack of resources.

Here it is interesting to note that economic incentives are attached to the work process of the Swedish nurses when they work with patients (see table 1). Nurses' documentation of their work with patients also means that information relating to the scope of the purchasing of services and setting targets is generated automatically. The primary care centre is evaluated in economic terms. For this reason, the purchaser – a political board – becomes the customer and consumer of health care, and not the individual patient. Consequently, the patient orientation of nurses as an economical tool is the capacity of nurses to behave competently in terms of the economic goals and standards of the purchaser and not in support of patients' recovery and wellbeing, a situation that is heavily criticised by the nurses.

REFERENCES

Allen, Davida (2004). Re-reading Nursing and Re-writing Practice: Towards an Empirically Based Reformulation of the Nursing Mandate. *Nursing Inquiry,* 11(4), 271-283.

An Bord Altranais (2000a). *Scope of Nursing and Midwifery Practice Framework.* Dublin: An Bord Altranais.

An Bord Altranais (2000b) *The Code of Professional Conduct for each Nurse and Midwife.* Dublin: An Bord Altranais.

Armstrong, D. (1998). The Fabrication of Nurse-Patient Relationships. In L Mackay, K. Soothill, and K. Melia. *Classic Texts in Health Care.* Oxford: Butterworth-Heinemann.

Beach, D. (Ed) (2005) *Work-package 2: Welfare State Restructuring in Education and Health Care: Implications for the Teaching and Nursing Professions and their Professional Knowledge.* Report no 2 from the PROFKNOW project. www.profknow.net

Bejerot, E. (2008). Patienten i centrum – ett tvingande styrningsideal. (The patient at the centre – a forcing governing ideal) In H. Hasselbladh, E. Bejerot, & R Å Gustafsson. B*ortom New Public Management – Institutionell transformation i svensk sjukvård.* (Beyond New Public Management - Institutional transformation in Swedish health care) Lund: Academia Adacta AB.

Björvell, C., Wredling, R. & Thorell-Ekstrand I. (2002). Long-term Increase in Quality of Nursing Documentation: Effects of a Comprehensive Intervention. *Scandinavian Journal of Caring Sciences,* 16(1), 34-42.

Blomgren, M. (2003). Ordering a Profession: Swedish Nurses Encounter New Public Management Reforms. *Financial Accountability & Management,* 19(1), 45-71.

Boerma, W.G.W. (2006). Coordination and Integration in European Primary Care. In R.B. Saltman, A. Rico, and W. Boerma (Eds.). *Primary Care in the Driver's Seat? Organizational Reform in European Primary Care.* Berkshire: McGraw-Hill Education. Open University Press.

Coulter, A. & Magee, H. (Eds.) (2003). *The European Patient of the Future.* Maidenhead: Open University Press.

de la Cuesta, C. (1983). The Nursing Process: From Development to Implementation. *Journal of Advanced Nursing,* 8, 36-371.

Dent, M., (2003) *Remodelling Hospitals and Health Professions in Europe*: Medicine, Nursing and the State, London: Palgrave Macmillan.

du Gay, P. & Salaman, JG. (1992). Enterprise culture and the search for "excellence"', *Sociologie et Societies,* 23 (2), 129-150.

Dupont, M. & Sugrue, C. (2007). Irish Nurses' Work and Life under Restructuring: Professional Experiences, Knowledge and Expertise in Changing Contexts. In T. Kosonen, & J. Houtsonen J. (Eds.) *European Nurses' Life and Work under Restructuring: Professional Experiences, Knowledge and Expertise in Changing Context.* Report no 5 from the PROFKNOW project. www.profknow.net

Ehnfors M., Thorell-Ekstrand I. & Ehrenberg A. (1991) Towards Basic Nursing Information in Patient Records. *Vård i Norden,* 21, 12–31.

Ehnfors, M., Ehrenberg, A. & Thorell-Ekstrand, I. (1998). *VIPS-boken: om en forskningsbaserad modell för dokumentation av omvårdnad i patientjournalen* (The VIPS-book: about a research modell for documentation of caring in the patient record). Stockholm: Vårdförb. SHSTF

Erickson, R.J. & Grove, W.J.C. (2008) Emotional Labor and Health Care. *Sociology Compass,* 2(2), 704-733.

Ehrenberg, A., Ehnfors, M. & Thorell-Ekstrand, I. (1996). Nursing Documentation in Patient Records: Experience of the Use of the VIPS model. *Journal of Advanced Nursing,* 24 (4), 853-867.

Figueras, J., McKee, M., Mossialos, E. & Saltman, R.B. (2003). Series Editors' Introduction. In *Regulating Entrepreneurial Behaviour in European Health Systems.* Buckingham Philadelphia: Open University Press.

Goodson, I. & Lindblad, S. (Eds.) (2008). *Cross-professional Studies on Nursing and Teaching in Europe.* Deliverable 6 in the EU Sixth Framework Programme Project Professional Knowledge in Education and Health: Restructuring Work and Life between the State and the Citizens in Europe. www.profknow.net

HSL 1982: 763 Swedish Heath Care Act. www.socialstyrelsen.se [Accessed August 1, 2008].

Kosonen, T. & Houtsonen, J. (Eds). (2007). *European Nurses' Life and Work under Restructuring: Professional Experiences, Knowledge and Expertise in Changing Context.* Report no 5 from the PROFKNOW project. www.profknow.net

Lannerholm, L. (1995). *Syster blir till: en sociologisk studie av sjuksköterskeyrkets framväxt och omformering* (Sister was born: a sociological study on the growing and transformation of the nurses occupation). Gothenburg: University of Gothenburg. Department of Sociology. Doctoral thesis.

Levin, M. (1971). Holistic Care. *The Nursing Clinics of North America*, 6(2), 253-264.

The National Board of Health and Welfare (2005). *Kompetensbeskrivning för legitimerad sjuksköterska* (Competence description for legitimate nurse). www.socialstyrelsen.se [Accessed August 1, 2008].

Roper, N. Logan, W. and Tierney, A. (1985). The Roper/Logan/Tierny model. *Senior Nurse*, 3(2), 20-26.

Saltman, R.B. (1992). *Patientmakt över vården*. (Patient-power over health care) Stockholm: SNS.

Saltman, R. B. (2002) Regulating Incentives: the Past and Present Role of the State in Health Care Systems. *Social Science & Medicine*, 54, 1677-1684.

Saltman, R.B., Busse, R. & Mossialos, E. (Eds.). (2002). *Regulating Entrepreneurial Behaviour in European Health Care Systems*. Buckingham, Philadelphia. Open University Press.

Saltman, R.B., Rico, A. and Boerma, W. (Eds.). (2006). *Primary Care in the Driver's Seat? Organizational Reform in European Primary Care*. Berkshire: McGraw-Hill Education. Open University Press.

Sen, K. (Ed). (2003). *Restructuring Health Services: Changing Contexts and Comparative Perspectives*. London: Zed Books.

Smith, P (1998). The Emotional Labour of Nursing: Its Impact on Interpersonal Relations, Management and the Educational Environment in Nursing. In L. Mackay, K. Soothill, and K. Melia. (Eds.). *Classic Texts in Health Care*. Oxford: Butterworth-Heinemann.

Vaartio, H. & Leino-Kilpi, H. (2005). Nursing Advocacy – a Review of the Empirical Research 1990-2003. *International Journal of Nursing Studies*, 42(6), 705-714.

Wärvik, G.-B. (2007). Nurses' Life Histories: The Swedish Case. In T. Kosonen & J. Houtsonen (Eds.) *European Nurses' Life and Work under Restructuring: Professional Experiences, Knowledge and Expertise in Changing Context*. Report no 5 from the PROFKNOW project. www.profknow.net

CONTRIBUTORS

Dennis Beach is Professor of Education at the University of Borås, Sweden, and visiting Professor at Roehampton University, London, England. His main research interests are the effects of restructuring in the welfare professions (particularly nursing, teaching and teacher education), education policy research, education and democracy, ethnography and the sociology of education. He is currently leading or involved in several national and international research projects in these fields or related areas. dennis.beach@hb.se

Magdalena Czaplicka is Licentiate of Philosophy at the Department of Social Work of Stockholm University, Sweden. Her main research focus is living conditions of youth, their political attitudes and activity. In addition, she has done research on literature for young people, especially young girls. During her research career she has produced about twenty articles and book chapters. Magdalena.Czaplicka@comhem.com

Maeve Dupont is Assistant Lecturer in the Special Education Department, St Patrick's College of Education, a college of Dublin City University, Ireland. Her most recent research activity is a project on the role of special schools and classes in Ireland. She is currently working on a research project addressing the challenges of inclusion in Irish schools. maeve.dupont@spd.dcu.ie

Rita Foss Lindblad got her PhD in Theory of Science and is a Senior Lecturer in Education at the University of Gothenburg, Sweden. Her research focuses on the social organisation of knowledge and learning in contemporary societies; of special interest are the political dimensions, where issues of gender, class, ethnicity and sexuality are important, as are issues of policies, educational systems and their epistemic configurations. At present she is investigating higher education and life-long learning, on the one hand, and professionalism, on the other hand. Her interests are motivated by their actuality and their complex linkage to the politics of education. rita.foss@ped.gu.se

Jarmo Houtsonen is Senior Researcher in the Department of Sociology and Social Policy at the University of Joensuu, Finland. He has published on education, culture and identity, contracting between business firms, and welfare state restructuring and schools. His research interests include institutions, economic sociology of law and research methods. jarmo.houtsonen@joensuu.fi

Toni Kosonen, BSc, is a Project Researcher in the Department of Sociology and Social Policy, University of Joensuu, Finland. His main areas of research are work and working life under restructuring and vocational education of low-skilled adults, more specifically questions concerning participation, access and outreach activities. toni.kosonen@joensuu.fi

Sverker Lindblad is Professor of Education at the University of Gothenburg, Sweden. He was one of the founders of the Nordic Educational Research Association and coordinator of the PROFKNOW project. He has also coordinated a European Union research project on Education Governance and Social Inclusion/Exclusion. Lindblad is doing research on international statistics and supra-national governing of education, e.g. in terms of comparative studies and ranking lists. In a similar manner he is now developing research on the politics of learning in classroom interaction. sverker.lindblad@ped.gu.se

Isaac Marrero, PhD, is a Researcher at the Centre for the Study of Changes in Culture and Education, University of Barcelona, Spain. For the past five years his main research focus has been the social, economic and physical transformation of Barcelona, the Poblenou neighbourhood in particular. A second area of research has been the politics of representation, an ongoing critical inquiry into the political dimension of the act of re-presenting. In broader terms, he is interested in the 'Post-Fordist transformation' of the relations of production and its impact in everyday life. He has specialized in ethnographic research. imarregu7@docd1.ub.edu

Jörg Müller, PhD in Communications, is a Researcher at the IN3 Internet Interdisciplinary Institute, Universitat Oberta de Catalunya (UOC), Spain. His main research interest is the impact of Information and Communication Technologies on society, especially the study of change in education and youth cultures. His theoretical interests are media theory, emotional and aesthetic dimensions of labour and communication. jmuller@uoc.edu

Helder Rocha Pereira is a PhD candidate at the Ponta Delgada Nursing School of the University of the Azores, Portugal. His main research focus is nursing and professional nursing care development related to facilitating transition processes of people with health/illness related problems, namely the understanding of transition experiences in respect to the role of an informal caregiver after unexpected events. Through the understanding of sudden caregiver experiences, it will be possible to determine key points in this transition process, define adequate nursing therapeutics and identify indicators allowing us to assess a successful transition. hpereira@uac.pt

Constantina Safiliou-Rothschild is Professor Emeritus at Wageningen Agricultural University, The Netherlands. She is a member of the Executive Committee of 50+Hellas, Greece. Her current research focuses on men's conditions, men in "feminine" stereotyped occupations and health and age discrimination. safiliou@otenet.gr

Peter Sohlberg is Professor in Sociology at Uppsala University and Senior Lecturer at the Department of Social Work at Stockholm University, Sweden. His main research focus is sociological theory and its empirical application, philosophy of science, and empirical studies of "epistemic cultures". peter.sohlberg@socarb.su.se

Gun-Britt Wärvik is Senior Lecturer at the Department of Education, University of Gothenburg, Sweden. Her research interest concerns political aspects of pedagogical phenomena, especially within the areas of lifelong learning and the politics of expertise. This includes the study of institutional change and governing technologies related to notions of performance and competence. gun-britt.warvik@ped.gu.se

www.ingramcontent.com/pod-product-compliance
Lightning Source LLC
Chambersburg PA
CBHW071348230926
51846CB00002B/479
9789087909802